Constructive Campaigning
for Autism Services

of related interest

Surviving the Special Educational Needs System
How to be a 'Velvet Bulldozer'
Sandy Row
ISBN 1 84310 262 5

Access and Inclusion for Children with Autistic Spectrum Disorders
'Let Me In'
Matthew Hesmondhalgh and Christine Breakey
ISBN 1 85302 986 6

Understanding Autism Spectrum Disorders
Frequently Asked Questions
Diane Yapko
ISBN 1 84310 756 2

Asperger's Syndrome
A Guide for Parents and Professionals
Tony Attwood
ISBN 1 85302 577 1

Constructive Campaigning for Autism Services

The PACE Parents' Handbook

Armorer Wason

Foreword by Virginia Bovell and Su Thomas

Jessica Kingsley Publishers
London and Philadelphia

First published in 2005
by Jessica Kingsley Publishers
116 Pentonville Road
London N1 9JB, UK
and
400 Market Street, Suite 400
Philadelphia, PA 19106, USA

www.jkp.com

Library of Congress Cataloging in Publication Data
Wason, Armorer, 1956-
    Constructive campaigning for autism services : the PACE parents' handbook / Armorer
Wason ; foreword by Virginia Bovell and Su Thomas.
        p. cm.
    Includes bibliographical references and index.
    ISBN-13: 978-1-84310-387-5 (pbk. : alk. paper)
    ISBN-10: 1-84310-387-7 (pbk. : alk. paper) 1. Autistic children--Services for--Great
Britain. 2. Autistic children--Education--Great Britain. 3. Autistic children--Rehabilita-
tion--Great Britain. 4. Parents of autistic children. I. Title.
    RJ506.A9W374 2005
    649'.154--dc22
                                    2005018074

British Library Cataloguing in Publication Data
A CIP catalogue record for this book is available from the British Library

ISBN 13: 978 1 84310 387 5
ISBN 10: 184310 387 7

Printed and bound in Great Britain by
Athenaeum Press, Gateshead, Tyne and Wear

Although every effort has been made to check the information contained in this book,
we cannot guarantee its accuracy, particularly given the pace of change in autism
and children's services. We would be grateful if any errors or inaccuracies could be
brought to our attention at handbook@treehouse.org.uk

It's all so tied up with my son. When he was first diagnosed, and I couldn't access anything, I couldn't find any information, I made him a small promise – that I would change the world.

– Helen Geldard, parent of a child with autism

TreeHouse: the national charity for autism education

TreeHouse, the national charity for autism education in the UK, was founded in 1997 by a group of parents of children with autism.

TreeHouse's vision is to transform through education the lives of children with autism and their families. It does this through its flagship school in north London, through working to support and empower professionals and parents across the country to expand the range of high-quality autism services, and through policy and campaigning.

The policy and campaigning work of TreeHouse is aimed at ensuring that autism is high on the agenda of decision-makers and opinion-formers, nationally and locally. The work has been consolidated through a merger with the charity PACE (formerly Parents Autism Campaign for Education) which took place in February 2005. PACE had already contributed to a range of government-sponsored materials and guidance on autism, and both charities had provided ongoing commentary, analysis and media coverage about the needs of children with autism. The merger has enabled this work to continue and expand.

TreeHouse is very keen to build alliances and partnerships across the autism movement. With the National Autistic Society it ran the first ever autism-specific campaign in a UK General Election during April 2005. It is also a member of the Advisory Group to the All Party Parliamentary Group on Autism, and collaborates with several other autism charities and parent groups, professionals, providers and academics, in order to make a difference for all children with autism.

Contact details:
The TreeHouse Trust
Woodside Avenue
London N10 3JA
General Enquiries: 020 8815 5444
School: 020 8815 5424
Facsimile: 020 8815 5420
Email: info@treehouse.org.uk
Website: www.treehouse.org.uk
Registered charity number 1063184
® TreeHouse is the registered trademark of the TreeHouse Trust

TreeHouse

Contents

Acknowledgements

The PACE Parents' Handbook has emerged from a rich collaboration with the co-directors of PACE: Virginia Bovell, one of the parent founders of PACE, brought a vision and understanding of policy, and a wealth of ideas from her campaigning experience. Steve Broach, policy consultant to the project, made an important contribution with his in-depth knowledge of policy development and legislation. Their support for the project has been unstinting.

Many thanks are also due to the parent trustees of PACE: Cathy Tissot, Hilarie Williams and in particular Su Thomas, the first chair of PACE, who pioneered taking a strategic approach to campaigning in her local authority.

I am grateful to Rebecca Simor for kick-starting the project with her initial research on the workings of local government, and to Chris Brierley for his cartoons. We were delighted that Jessica Kingsley Publishers agreed to publish the Handbook, and we are particularly grateful to Jessica herself for her encouragement and constructive editorial advice.

The book could not have been researched and written without the support of Lloyds TSB Foundation, and PACE is very grateful for the commitment of Jude Stevens to the success of the project. PACE is also grateful for donations from Abel Hadden, ARM Ltd, Cable and Wireless plc, Scottish Power and Weber Shandwick.

The Handbook draws on in-depth discussions with experienced parent campaigners, and with professionals and public authority officers who have developed strong and effective relationships with parents and parent groups. It has also benefited from discussions with a number of local and national politicians and civil servants, who have given a great deal of time and thought to the contents.

In particular I would like to thank Sharon Bradbroke-Armit, Christine Bowker, Pat Cherry, Patience Cobley, Michael Dishington, Catherine Gee, Esther Fletcher, Jeremy Fordham, Vicky Foreman, Helen Geldard, Philip and Chareline Gibbs, Peter Gurney, Astrid Hansen, Kevin Healey, Carol Kelsey, Claire le Feuvre, Stella Mabb, Sheila Moorcroft, Liz Morris, Kevin O'Byrne, Susie O'Kelly, Pamela Reitemeier, Philippa Shipley, Sam Silver and Sara Truman.

Many colleagues in autism and other children's and disability voluntary sector organisations have taken the time to comment on drafts. PACE is very grateful to Colin Barrow, Francine Bates, Amanda Batten, Angie Lee-Foster, Brendan King, Christine Lenehan, Margaret McGowan, David Potter, Carol Povey, Carole Rutherford, Pauline Shelley and Alison Tarrant for constructive and thoughtful feedback.

I would also like to express our thanks to the many parents, professionals, politicians and civil servants who have made highly valued contributions to the Handbook, but have requested that we do not acknowledge them by name.

Armorer Wason
May 2005

Foreword

We never meant to lobby or campaign, any more than we meant to have children with autism. We certainly never thought that there might one day be a handbook arising from our experiences – alongside that of hundreds of other parents who similarly found themselves turning into unexpected campaigners. But anyone who has had a child with a disability is forced into a world where life takes unexpected turns, a world in which the desire to make a difference for your own child is joined by a desire to make a difference for others in similar situations.

This book is therefore for all parents of children with autism, including those who, like us, may not see themselves as natural campaigners. It is rooted in the experiences of parents who have made a difference, and we hope it will be an inspiration for those of you who are just starting out.

We didn't know at the time it was campaigning. We thought it was discussing with, cajoling and persuading local authority officers to recognise that there was a gap in children's autism services. We could see that this gap could only be met through strategic means – planning ahead, investing, innovating – rather than sticking on the treadmill of out-dated prevalence rates, low educational standards and low professional expectations. We then started doing exactly the same things at national level – discussing and cajoling and persuading, armed this time with statistics, knowledge of the current policy climate and arguments that we hoped would resonate with decision-makers.

Some people don't think of themselves as campaigners because it sounds aggressive and even military. Indeed, many parents of children with autism, as with many other disabilities, have said they feel they are in a war zone – both in terms of the fight they are undergoing for their children but also in terms of the solidarity they feel with other parents in similar battles. We have felt similarly at times. However, we also want to explain and translate this experience so that people who are outside the war zone, or who are unaware they are in it, can understand. Permanent war is exhausting and destructive; we need to find alternative ways of ensuring that children with autism don't get short-changed. Only when an inspirational mother (quoted in this book) from County Durham went to her dictionary and found that to campaign is to 'take an organised course of action' did we feel completely sure that this is the word to describe the work that needs to be done.

PACE was set up as an umbrella for all the separate parent initiatives that existed at the time to improve access to crucial education for children with autism. Between 1997 and 2005 we have talked with and heard from thousands of parents all over the UK, we have sat on local government and national working parties and groups, and we have seen new initiatives on autism spring up from the growing awareness among decision-makers that autism isn't going to go away.

The first stage in the 'campaign' has been achieved. Awareness of autism is greater, at parliamentary and national government level. But what is really crucial is the second stage. Greater awareness does not automatically translate into improved services. Recent government initiatives outlined in this book are a genuine step forward but this doesn't mean they are enough. And they will mean very little unless they take root up and down the country. This is what this book is about. Now is a crucial time – we need to ensure that the central initiatives really do mean something on the ground for children with autism. Parents really *can* make a difference by holding local agencies to account and by bringing their experience to the table, so that all the good words expressed by politicians can mean something real for children throughout the country.

In this book, we want to offer a resource to parents, based on the experiences and achievements of other parents, to help you decide the best way to approach your local authority when pursuing the goal of better services for all children. We hope you will read it and see where you feel you might fit in.

As for us, there are still times when it feels like being in a war, but in reality it is a journey with great highs and lows. Along the way we have developed great friendships, met inspirational people. And the highest highs of all are those occasions when we hear from other parents who have really made a difference to their children and to the lives of other children in their area. A local success offers inspiration everywhere. Keep going! And if possible we hope you enjoy the journey...

Virginia Bovell and Su Thomas
PACE founding parents

1. Introduction

What is the Parents' Handbook?

This handbook is first and foremost for parents who want to play a key role in developing better services for children with autism.[1] It is rooted in the experiences of parents who have done this, and offers insights based on what their campaigning has achieved to date.[2] It may also be useful to parents seeking to improve services for children with other disabilities, or to campaigners who want to achieve better support for adults with disabilities, not least those adults themselves. And last but not least, it may help public authority officers to develop their work with parents.

Parents have a crucial role to play in raising the standards of autism service provision. We know from talking to parents just how much can be achieved through their skills, energies and passion. And we have learnt that there are particular things parents need to know to ensure that their campaigning is fully effective.

This handbook therefore provides the background information about local authority structures and government policy which will help with effective campaigning. It is built on the real-life experiences of parents who between them have adopted a range of approaches to influencing local agencies, and who speak for themselves in the extensive quotations throughout this book. We talked in depth to many individual parents throughout England and Wales, and to members of over 20 parents' groups in north-east England, south-west England, the Midlands, inner and outer London, the Home Counties and south Wales.

---

1   Throughout this text, the term 'autism' has been used as shorthand for all conditions on the autistic spectrum, including Asperger syndrome. Where we refer exclusively to specific conditions such as Asperger syndrome, we make this clear in the text.
2   Throughout the text, all unattributed quotations are from parents of children with autism who are campaigning for better autism services.

We also talked to officers in local agencies and government civil servants, and to local and national politicians, to get a broader view.

Much of the focus of our work has been on education, as this is often the key service for children with ASDs (autism spectrum disorders) and their families. But increasingly education, health and social services are overlapping; this handbook looks at how parents can influence all relevant agencies in a changing world.

What is PACE?

PACE was founded and run by parents of children with autism, working locally and nationally across England and Wales to improve autism services. Since February 2005, PACE has been the policy and campaigns team of TreeHouse, the national charity for autism education. We make recommendations to national government based on parents' experiences, give advice to parents on local lobbying, and put parents in touch with advocacy organisations that can help them with individual casework.

Working for all children with autism

Parents who fight for services for their own children and families quickly come up against the scale of the system's failure to deliver appropriate or sufficient services. If parents manage to access what their child and family needs, they are only too aware that the majority cannot get the same deal. So this handbook is about the next step: it is for parents who want to put effort into building better services for ALL children with autism.

Not surprisingly, many of these parents are put off by the Alice-in-Wonderland world of local government, the attitudes of hard-pressed professionals or an understandable scepticism about whether anything they do will lead to real change. So...

...Why get involved?

Every time I drive past the school that has come out of our work I feel a real sense of pride. If you begin to get a sense of achievement, you begin to feel more in control, more effective, and your stress levels are reduced.

The involvement of parents makes a real difference to the quality of services. Parents have a unique and vital understanding of what 'good services' should look like. Only parents can bring an authoritative perspective on the genuine needs, as opposed to the perceived needs, of children and families.

> The multi-agency review (a major consultation with parents and children with disabilities) threw up some surprises. Officers had predicted that more residential respite care was needed, but it became apparent that a whole range of services was necessary, and that if they were in place, residential services would in fact be less necessary.

Parents can build bridges and break through professional silos, providing moral authority to force professionals to talk to each other. Sometimes this is done through skilled informal networking by parents, who are likely to come into contact with a range of different professionals in different agencies.

> Having a finger in every pie means that often you know much more than the professionals do about what's going on. You can say, 'but I was at a meeting with so-and-so last week and this has already been discussed...'

> We ran a training day on Asperger syndrome with the focus on bringing together professionals from different agencies to work together. After a very good range of presentations we divided people into cross-agency groups so that everyone was new to each other, and gave them a problem that they could only solve by working together. We had fantastic feedback. People really valued working with other agencies, making contacts, developing practical strategies and gaining a new understanding of the issue.

Professionals can find it hard to see beyond bureaucratic constraints. Parents can help them to cut through to what really matters.

> Parents can ask the simple but really important questions that can actually move everyone on. You can interrupt our jargon and fixed ideas, and help us think through our assumptions. (Local authority officer)

There are also indirect benefits for parents and their families that some people have found very valuable.

> It has brought rewards for the whole family. We've got to know so many other families, we've created a community. If you can stop

another parent from going through what you've been through, it brings something positive out of something very hard.

Parents can inspire councillors and officers at all levels to 'champion' the interests of children with autism.

The key is to find just one person who wants to help. It makes all the difference to find a mover in the system.

This is crucially important. The Audit Commission's (2003) report, *Services for Disabled Children*, states:

It seems that disabled children get on the agenda if local champions put them there, but are at risk of tumbling back down if these champions move on. (p.10)

You don't always have to make your views known: you can be effective through being a persistent presence. Sometimes just turning up at a meeting and reminding professionals that parents exist is worthwhile.

We didn't know when we sat quietly through endless meetings talking about the plumbing in a vacant health centre room that it would one day lead to a thriving family resource centre – instinct just told us to keep going to the meetings and to remind everyone that the room had been earmarked for parents.

And you may even feel you've made a real mess of it – but you might be surprised.

My sole contribution to my first meeting was with the leader of the council was to pour coffee into the tea-pot… Nobody laughed and I wanted to die. But three years later the (now ex-) leader of the council supported our case and his support helped swing it for us.

Parents might feel deterred in the short term, but it is important not to give up. Changing how public organisations work does take time, particularly when aiming for meaningful and sustainable change. Policy or provision that is based on panic rarely works well. Frustration over timescales is often shared by service providers. As one local authority officer stated:

It is hard to understand why change is so slow. It's not to do with lack of will, but about how complex it is to make change happen. It's easy to say, we don't have a school, why don't we just open a unit? But it's much more complicated than that. We find it frustrating too. (Local authority officer)

It's worth remembering that fifty years ago there was no provision for children with autism. Parents were blamed for the condition, and all society had to offer was long-stay institutional care and inappropriate medication. It is thanks to the people who were wrongly described as 'failed bonders' or 'refrigerator mothers' and to their enlightened professional allies, that society now recognises that our children are entitled to more appropriate and autism-sensitive interventions. We are still a long way off from meeting the needs of all children with autism, but never doubt the power that parents have in accelerating the pace of change.

Why get involved now?

Since the National Autistic Society (NAS) was founded by parents over 40 years ago, parents have led the way at every stage in developing decent services for children with autism. Yet there has never been a better time for parent activism than right now.

Through the Children's National Service Framework (NSF), a set of standards for children's services, the Government has now officially recognised the vital role that parents can play in implementing policy at local level, and driving forward improvements to services:

> Listening to the views of parents is one of the most effective ways of improving support services for them... Involvement of children and their parents in planning services results in the provision of more appropriate services. (Department of Health and Department for Education and Skills 2004a, p.29, p.84)

The NSF view of parent activism is supported by a number of other key initiatives in recent years (see Chapter 9 for more information about these policy initiatives):

- The children's green paper *Every Child Matters* (2003a) creates a framework for the whole of children's services which recognises the important role of parents as equal partners with professionals and service providers.

- The government-sponsored *Autistic Spectrum Disorders Good Practice Guidance* (Department for Education and Skills/Department of Health 2002) shows parents exactly what an 'autism- friendly' school or local educational authority (LEA) might look like, and again emphasises partnership with parents.

Parents who have been involved in translating these initiatives into action have seen real improvements.

> Every Child Matters *and the* National Service Framework *have hit the nail on the head. Now professionals who have the will to do something about the problems have a legitimate reason to go ahead. Our county was in the dark ages, but in twelve months it has developed into a 'cutting edge' authority.*

Local authorities, primary care trusts and other agencies will be inspected against the NSF standards, which in time should lead to improvements to services. However, parental pressure is vital to ensure that the NSF standards are prioritised and therefore implemented quickly and in full by local public agencies.

> *My experience is that the authority is painfully aware of the new national government initiatives, you don't need to tell them what they are. The best way in is to say, 'we know there's no magic wand or pot of gold, but can we help you to implement these?'.*

The law is also changing in ways that support improvements to autism services. Schools and local education authorities have new legal planning duties that require them to make their services progressively more accessible to all disabled people (see Department for Education and Skills 2002). Recent additions to the Disability Discrimination Act mean that all public bodies, including schools, are required to promote equality of opportunity for disabled people. This is potentially a very powerful tool for campaigners: commentators recognise that the equivalent duty with regard to race equality has been the most significant catalyst for improvements in this area.

Yet although the current legal and policy climate supports positive change, the danger is that if parents don't get involved, the postcode lottery of provision will continue, as only the 'good' authorities set about improving their services in line with government guidelines.

Differences between LEAs: 'customised campaigning'

How parents go about campaigning for better autism services will vary according to local conditions. One of the most important conditions will be the attitude of local agencies to working with parents. More enlightened and forward-thinking authorities will recognise that involving parents will help them do their job better – providing effective services and meeting their legal responsibilities to their clients. In these authorities, parents will be able to work with councillors, officers and others to maximise the chances that services will genuinely improve. Guidance on how parents can best achieve this is set out in Chapters 3 and 5.

Other agencies may pay lip service to consultation, but may not be willing or able to follow through with real improvements, or even to take parents seriously. In these situations, parents may choose to persevere with efforts to develop genuine collaboration, but will need to assess their progress carefully over time. This is when the lobbying methods discussed at the end of Chapter 5 and in Chapter 6 can be considered. These methods may be particularly appropriate when parents have to defend existing services from cuts or closures – something which may have to take place before efforts to develop a more positive dialogue with professionals about service improvement can begin.

It is vital to recognise that 'good' and 'bad' authorities are not set in stone. How authorities work with parents and provide services will be subject to changes in personnel, funding and policy (both national and local). Power may shift between levels of the system, for instance from local education authorities to schools. The message here is that parents need to be flexible in their relationship with authorities, picking the most appropriate strategies to use at any particular time.

Parents who make a commitment to learning how things work locally have managed to have real influence and bring about real change. Parent action in one local authority resulted in a major review of autism services and a decision to allocate dedicated funds each year to early intervention home programmes. This is just one of hundreds of examples where parents have brought about tangible improvements to services, transforming the lives of children with autism. That is why campaigning matters – and in the chapters that follow we outline how to make sure your efforts are most effective.

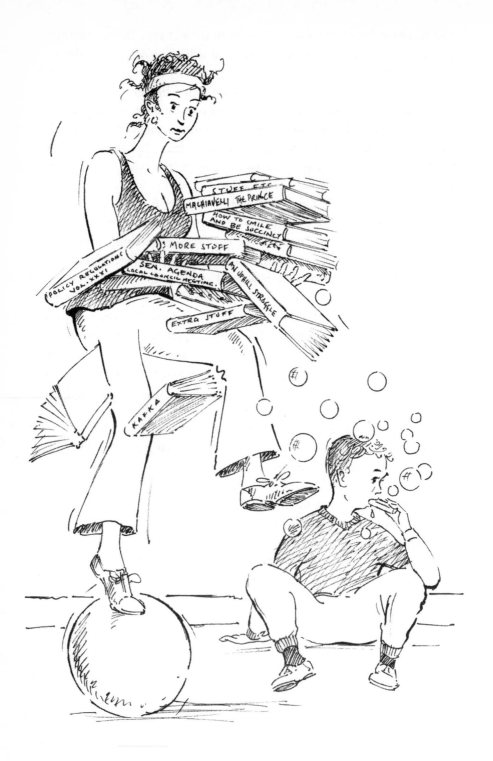

2. Before you begin… [1]

PACE's view of successful campaigning is that it must be 'customised'. By this we mean that there are no universal right answers in terms of what works, but only approaches suited to particular conditions. At the end of the day, autism campaigners have to convince people with power to do things better. Genuine influence relies on calm and persistent communication of parental experiences to the right people, at the right time and in the right ways. If the only thing that people remember about you is that you are angry, you are unlikely to achieve long-term change.

To be effective, parents need to be able to step back from their emotions and calmly consider their objectives in the light of local conditions, personalities and other factors. By doing this, they will be able to choose the approach that is most likely to work in their particular situation, and at the particular stage that they have reached in the process. We are not suggesting that parents need to detach themselves from their emotions – clearly, this is impossible. But we do need to recognise that raw emotion rarely, if ever, strengthens our case.

Separating two objectives: improving services for all children with autism and seeking to meet your own child's needs

In retrospect I think that trying to raise issues to do with provision when we were all trying to secure appropriate schooling for our own children was just too hard.

Experienced parent campaigners stress the importance of separating the two struggles – fighting for their own child on the one hand, and

---

1   Throughout this chapter we refer to organisations and documents. Please see the Resources section at the end of the book for more information about how to contact and access these materials.

working for a better deal for all children with autism on the other. Although not impossible, they feel that it is particularly difficult to work towards both these objectives at the same time.

> It's very hard not to get emotional or sucked into thinking only about your own child, but it is essential that you don't. I only turned to campaigning once I had sorted things out for my own child. It's no good bringing things up in the wrong forum – it doesn't help the policy discussion if you do it there, and it doesn't help you – you end up feeling frustrated, bitter, and deadlocked.

In any meeting or group set up to look at provision as a whole, it is essential that parents focus on the bigger picture, and put aside personal interests. Parents will not have impact if they are perceived to be 'one issue' campaigners – particularly if the issue in question affects solely or predominantly their own child.

> I was at a meeting of a small group of parents with an LEA official, trying to convince him that most ASD parents were against a policy of closing learning disability primary schools. It went really well until we were talking about the possibility of having an ASD-specific unit attached to a mainstream school, and when asked where would be best, one parent said, 'my son's school'. She gave no indication that this was for any other reason than to meet her own child's needs. I could tell that from then on, we would not be taken seriously – and we weren't.

Parents working with their local authority will find themselves in meetings with the same officers whom they talk to on other occasions purely about their own child's needs. This can require some delicate handling. Time constraints may tempt parents to raise individual issues at such meetings, but even when time is short, you should find a way to deal with the issues separately.

Keeping individual interests to one side in policy discussions is especially difficult when there is conflict over an individual case. One parent who has a significant role in policy discussions in her authority now faces real dilemmas about how to do this effectively while also taking her case to Tribunal. Another parent in a similar position managed to tackle the difficulty by making a point of explicitly recognising the potential for problems to officers:

> I told [the officer] 'We may have to go to Tribunal, but I want you to know that I believe in what the LEA is trying to do in lots of ways, even

if I have a separate disagreement about my child.' The officer accepted this and we both managed to keep the issues separate when we sat on the same advisory group.

However, it can be appropriate and helpful to draw on your own experience to illustrate a general point (see the section on 'Making an effective case: presentation skills' in Chapter 5, p.56).

Parents who have made headway with their local authorities are united in the view that the more they have managed to keep their feelings out of discussions with the local authorities, the more effective their efforts have been. These parents are in no doubt as to the difficulty that this can present:

Parents need to acknowledge that their grief gets in the way of things. It's so traumatic having a child with autism that you never get a chance to recover from the initial shock and pain of what has happened to your family. You're in post-traumatic shock, but you've no chance to deal with that, because you're dealing with the very real immediate issues of diagnosis, education, respite, their lack of awareness of danger...

And the challenge faced by parents is exacerbated by what is at stake:

The problem is that we're so emotionally involved – this is our children's future.

In the circumstances it is hardly surprising that it is difficult to engage dispassionately and constructively in policy discussions. Our advice is for parents to recognise what, realistically, they are able to take on. This will depend on where they are in the process of meeting their own child's needs. It is much easier to keep your emotional response out of the professional arena if your own child's needs are being met.

On the plus side, parents who do succeed in keeping their emotional response and individual interests to one side can be highly influential campaigners.

It isn't fair but keep an eye on your anger. You've every reason to moan but recognise that showing your feelings is unlikely to help, and that you will achieve much more if you don't. You have huge moral authority when, as a parent, you keep it together.

Working out what you want to achieve

Parents set out on the road of engagement with local authorities for a range of reasons.

- Some know exactly what they want to achieve – a specific goal such as a new unit or a new short-break service.
- Some wish to see general improvements locally – better communication with parents or speedier assessments.
- Others are less clear about the specifics, but just want to make local public agencies aware of the needs of families.

None of these are right or wrong, though it may be helpful for parents to clarify which category they fall into, since this may affect how they get started. But don't worry – it is not necessary to have it all worked out in advance.

Working with other parents

There are huge benefits in setting up or joining an existing parents' group, whether it is a group specifically for parents of children with autism, or a pan-disability group.

> Having a group that's in contact with a lot of other parents is a great mechanism for communicating parents' views anonymously to the public authorities.

It's good to have other parents to check ideas out with, to plan with, and for support.

Working in a group means that there is less pressure to throw yourself in at the deep end. Different parents will play different roles at different times. Making autism services better is a marathon, not a sprint. Parents who work as a group are able to choose priorities, share the work, and pace themselves.

Groups can have far more impact than parents working on their own. If you can demonstrate that you are in touch with a very broad range of parents beyond an 'inner circle', your group will gain legitimacy in the eyes of public authorities.

> Our local authority understands that working with us is a cost-effective way of getting it right. We have developed an 'information base' from the 240 paid-up members on our database. When the local public authorities ask for parents' views we send out a questionnaire and produce a report based on the feedback. Parents have seen results from this process and are very motivated to respond, and the authorities respect what we do.

What makes a group succeed as a group?

Several parents described problems they had encountered:

> The trouble is that when [X] is there, none of the rest of us can get a word in. What should we do when one person dominates discussion?'

> I've learned that when I'm talking about my own experience, I need to ask myself, 'Am I having a moan, or am I drawing on it to make a constructive point?' The former is definitely not helpful in a campaigning group.

> I spent two years doing everything. I had a real problem delegating, and looking back, I'm glad I did it, but I'm not sure we're that much further ahead.

Being alert to these potential problems will help avoid them becoming entrenched, as will awareness of the kinds of skills and abilities that make campaigning groups run well:

> Someone who keeps an overview of what needs doing, and when.

> People who help with things like distributing the newsletter, and licking envelopes.

> Someone who understands that groups need to be a bit stormy at times while they work things out, and that they usually come through the better for it.

> Someone who is a peacemaker, a negotiator; someone with a calming influence.

> Someone who is committed to working in and between meetings to ensure that the group's goals are met.

Several parents emphasise the importance of pulling together as a group, and of finding ways to manage disagreement and overcome difference.

> It doesn't make sense for individuals to follow their own agenda. We've recognised that the interests of the group are our own interests. We're much more effective working as a group.

Good communications are central to operating successfully and ensuring your reputation, both with the public authorities and with other parents. Regular meetings, newsletters and e-mail are good ways of communicating with group members.

> Parents feel lied to unless the information channels are open.

Before representing a group opinion to local public authorities, it is important that the parent concerned is genuinely informed of parents' views, and that the group has agreed any necessary policy positions in advance of meetings. Afterwards the parent should make sure that feedback is clearly given to all members: if parents are not told what is happening they may feel marginalised or ignored.

Bringing parents together to form a campaigning group
Exclusion is an issue for parents as well as for children with autism, and most groups are likely to benefit from efforts to reach out beyond the founding parents' immediate circle.

> We decided to have a formal constitution to be more organised and attract other parents. We've been holding our meetings in a local pub in the hope that that will feel accessible.

If you are not already in touch with local parents, you can use helplines like those run by organisations such as Contact a Family and the National Autistic Society (NAS) and also your local parent partnership service, to find out about parents and parent groups that may be active in your area.[2] PARIS (www.info.autism.org.uk), the online database run by the NAS, has a comprehensive list of all local autism groups.

Some parents have found it hard to find others to work with. If there is not an existing group of parent campaigners, parents' groups that currently concentrate on mutual support, social events or advice-giving might want to develop local campaigning work.

Some parents are justifiably anxious that they do not have the time or resources to offer very much. It may be a case of dipping your toe in the water and gradually getting more involved.

> Recognise that some parents will find this kind of work too demanding. Look for the parents who will enjoy it, the ones who see that they will get something out of it, who will see that it might add to the work they do: that it combats feelings of uselessness, knowing that what you're doing will improve the lives of many families.

And small contributions can in themselves be very helpful.

---

2   The work of parent partnership services is described on p.39.

The best support is from parents turning up to what we do, and turning up unasked to offer bits of help. And it really helps to be appreciated. When a thank you card comes in or Jo Bloggs who runs a pub does some fundraising, that really drives you on.

Parents may fear that getting involved will mean that they risk antagonising the very people on whom they and their child depend. There may be a basis for these feelings, but it is possible to come up with ways to protect individuals who express such concerns. Such parents may be able to provide valuable behind-the-scenes assistance – anything from Internet research to providing refreshments at a meeting – without needing to publicise their involvement.

There are times when we may all feel discouraged, even to believing that there is just no point in trying to change things. This can happen if change is taking a long time to achieve, or if improvements in services seem small compared with all that needs to be done, or if we are just exhausted. In these cases, it is amazing how helpful it can be to contact other parents who have seen things change over time as a result of their efforts, and whose own experiences show that getting involved really does work.

I decided I would drop out of the group for a while because I had so much on my plate. But very soon after that I got inspired again by hearing of a new initiative that I knew our group could respond to really easily, and meeting other parents who were really fired up about it.

Thinking long-term

It helps to think about the sustainability of your group as early as possible – because it is unlikely to be needed merely in the short term.

Think about succession planning – finding and supporting the person who is going to do your job when you no longer want to do it. Don't block other people coming forward. My predecessors found it quite hard to make way for me. You have to learn to let go and step back a bit, if you don't want this to be your life's work.

Alternatively, if you know that you can only offer a fixed period of your time, recognise this and deliberately aim for something short-term.

Even if you feel it slows you down, it is worth putting energy into bringing in and developing the skills of new parents.

Between the two of us we had a range of skills and achieved a lot very quickly, but it would have been much better if there had been more of us. We wouldn't have achieved so much so fast, but we would have built more of a base.

What degree of formality?

Groups can get a long way without having a formal organisational structure, particularly if they are clear about who does what. Some groups have found it useful if individual parents agree to take responsibility for a particular area – attending particular meetings, developing knowledge and contacts in a particular area of interest, or running a phone line, for instance. And one parent can take a lead role, checking overall progress and ensuring that decisions are made and stuck to.

But formal structures can be extremely helpful in giving authority and sustainability to the work done by groups of parents. Having a formal committee means that you ensure there is a body that is accountable for the organisation, and a formal mechanism for decision-making. Some may go further, and become a charitable trust involving a range of people as trustees beyond the initial parents:

Trustees can bring an outward view, which is vital, because you're up to your neck in it, living what your group is trying to achieve and sometimes that means that you cannot see the whole picture, or what other families need.

Where money is involved in particular, groups may want to adopt a formal constitution and think about acquiring charitable status.

We found that having charitable status definitely helped us open doors. The pack from the Charity Commission is very good, and they help you through the process.

Some groups have found it helpful to become a local branch of a national charity, such as the National Autistic Society or Contact a Family (see 'Advisory organisations and contact details' in the Resources section).

The NAS logo has helped us through the door with the local authority.

Having long-term impact as a group

For a campaigning group to have long-term impact, it helps to look at what skills and interests will be helpful, and who might have them, or be able to develop them.

Parents suggested the following:

Confidence with public speaking.

Someone who enjoys reading up about policy.

Analytical skills – someone who can see the big picture.

Being able to put your point of view across briefly and tactfully.

Someone who can write clearly, and who has basic research skills.

Someone who's not easily deterred, who can bring people together and open doors.

Parents who are persistent, who are prepared to attend meetings and keep tabs on things.

Someone who knows how important it is to keep other parents informed.

This list may seem formidable, but many parents have enjoyed building on skills and experience transferred from other areas of their lives, or developing new skills that they hadn't had an opportunity to discover before.

It is worth thinking carefully about who should represent the group to the public authorities. Often the right person is the parent who is the most convincing and diplomatic, and this is not necessarily the leading parent, or the person with the most passion.

Local authority officers describe attributes they value in parent representatives: 'the ability to look at the issues in the wider context'; 'an ability to do and reflect on research'; 'sensitivity to the people they're talking to'; 'ability to listen and build real dialogue'; 'someone with endurance, time and the personality to achieve the tasks'.

Parents agree that what really matters is the ability to relate to professionals.

You don't have to be posh, you can be dead ordinary. But you do have to go about things the right way.

Don't worry if you feel your group doesn't have the necessary skills. There are many organisations that provide advice, support and training to local voluntary groups. The Contact a Family/Council for Disabled Children (CDC/CaF) (2004) guide, *Parent Participation – Improving Services for Disabled Children*, is an invaluable manual (see below at the end of this chapter). You could also ask at your local library or contact the Council for Voluntary Service (see NACVS in the Resources section, p.108).

What are public authorities and services like in your area?

There is huge variation in the quality and quantity of services for children with autism across England and Wales. It is a good idea to find out something about the breadth of provision in your area before you start campaigning, even if you have a particular interest such as early intervention or a particular school. It is unlikely that you will be able to tell exactly what the agencies in your area are like until you start working with them. But whatever information you gain behind the scenes will be useful when you start approaching officers and councillors.

Local authorities have an obligation to make appropriate provision for the children in their area, and they should be looking ahead at shifts in need and demand, but there is no obligation on them to make a special study of a particular issue. Because of this, you may be surprised how little information there is on autism in your area.

There are acknowledged weaknesses in publicly collected statistics; the PLASC[3] data for instance, collected by schools, gives the numbers of children with a diagnosis of autism in an authority who are in school and getting additional support, but not the numbers of pre-school children, excluded children, or those who do not have a confirmed diagnosis or those not getting additional support. In this situation, parents have a valuable role in ensuring that deficiencies in information are pointed out in as non-critical a way as possible, and in requesting that decision-makers clarify the information base for specific policy decisions.

Information can be found in public authority development plans, which may be available to the public, and in public reports on how the authority spends its funding, but this may be very technical and complex. Some regions have attempted to map local need against provision. Where information is poor, you can suggest working together with the local authority to establish the facts. If you can develop a good mechanism for researching a problem collaboratively, you can remove a great deal of conflict from your discussions.

---

3   Pupil Level Annual School Census, which from 2004 has autistic spectrum disorder as a specific category.

The Department for Education and Skills (DfES) *Autism Spectrum Disorders Good Practice Guidance* (2002), mentioned on p.17, is a very useful audit tool. It is being used in some local authorities by parents and professionals to evaluate what is provided for children with ASD and to highlight areas that might need improving.

There is a wide range of information about local agencies, and much is available on the Internet. Your council should have a website, as should your primary care trust, strategic health authority, and DfES Special Educational Needs Regional Partnership.[4] If you can't find these sites through a search engine such as Google, you can ask the information officer at the local council for details. At www.upmystreet.com, you can type in your postcode and get the full range of contact details for your council – click on 'My council and reps' and scroll down to the 'Contacting your council' section.

Most council business is done in public. The agenda of meetings, working papers and minutes of meetings are all available and should be given to you free of charge. Local libraries hold copies of the dates, agenda and minutes of full council and committee meetings. Most authorities also publish them on their websites. The public has the legal right to attend meetings of the council and overview and scrutiny committees, except during discussion of exempt business, such as the care of a particular child.

Questions to inform your research

- How does your authority communicate with parents?

- Does support for children with autism seem to be of roughly the same standard, or are there particular areas or types of services that are much stronger or weaker than others?

- Are there other groups of parents of children with autism that are working with local public authorities, or perhaps a pan-disability parents' group? If so, what have they done? What is their focus, who do they mainly talk to? How do

4   DfES Special Educational Needs Regional Partnerships are structures that seek to improve SEN servicess by bringing agencies from local authorities together within each region. See www.teachernet.gov.uk/wholeschool/sen/regional

they see the problems? What do they make of local officers and the local council?

- What is your local authority's special educational needs (SEN) policy? Does it have an autism section? (It should be on the local authority website.)

- What is your LEA's record in going to the SEN and Disability Tribunal (SENDIST). This information is at the back of the SENDIST Annual Report.

- If the problems lie within your child's school, do you know how SEN is funded within your local authority? To what extent are funds delegated to schools? If they have been delegated, what accountability mechanisms, if any, have been put into place to monitor how children with SEN fare under delegated funding?

Learning how agencies plan future services

As you develop knowledge of the problems within your authority, you may also take an interest in the structures for developing services for autism. One of the most useful things to learn is how agencies in your area plan future services. The Audit Commission (2003) report on disabled children's services stated that strategic planning is hampered by a lack of four basic building blocks (p.15):

- *An understanding of the level of need*: 'neither commissioners nor providers had a comprehensive understanding of the numbers of local disabled children…or the type or complexity of their needs'.

- *Comprehensive knowledge of what services are available*: 'We did not find any examples of a whole-systems review of services being carried out to identify gaps and overlaps or to look at effective resource use'.

- *A clear picture of finance, costs and resources*: 'Many services could not supply accurate cost information for the client group'.

- *Strong inter-agency relationships*: 'Strategic planning was often disrupted by local structural changes in services that had been carried out as a result of national policy'.

Do you get the impression that your local agencies have the knowledge and relationships described above, or the commitment to put resources into developing these?

Very few, if any, authorities would claim to have got everything right for children with autism. It is important to keep an open mind about the problems, and not to confuse impact with intention. Don't assume that poor services or poor planning are always the result of wilful obstructiveness or that decisions are 'stitched up' by local officers. Often the cause of these barriers is institutional rather than individual, perhaps coupled with a lack of awareness about the particular needs of children with autism. Parents can play a huge part in addressing both these problems.

You may have to keep reminding your authority of the importance of handling communication with parents with utmost care, and that if they do not, they run the risk of seeming callous or indifferent, in which case genuine attempts to bring about improvements to services will be met with cynicism. Authorities that truly seek to bring about change need to develop the skills to bring parents and service-users along with them, ideally through a sophisticated communication process which ensures that parents are properly involved from the outset. This might be something that you could help your authority develop.

The issues to consider before you begin may seem daunting, but you don't need to have everything in place before you approach the authorities. How you might go about this is tackled in the next chapter.

A publication that is likely to be very helpful both to you and to the professionals you are working with is *Parent Participation – Improving Services for Disabled Children*, available from Contact a Family. It takes the form of two guides, one for parents and one for professionals (see 'Advisory organisations and contact details' in the Resources section).

3. Initial steps in approaching public authorities

Thinking around the problems

Nick Hornby, parent of a child with autism, addressed the Labour Party conference in 2003 on the structural difficulties faced by parents:

> What has shocked me most in my experience as the father of a disabled child is the inescapable sense that many of the professionals that parents have to deal with on a daily basis are regarded as the enemy... Now, we are talking here about people who presumably went into their profession because they are motivated by a desire to care and help, to serve the public; what they end up doing is obstructing and delaying and frustrating the parents of the most vulnerable members of our society, disabled children. I don't believe that these people are bad, so what is going on here?

As parents we don't get to pick the officers who will control budgets and policy decisions in our local agencies. We have to work with who is there. However, there are two important things to recognise:

1. It is always worth remembering that behind an obstructive individual officer lies an inflexible system that may well have worn that person down over a number of years (see Chapter 10). As far as possible, we think it makes more sense to re-ignite the enthusiasm of professionals and local officers, than to make their jobs even more pressurised.

    PACE believes that the most effective way forward for parent campaigners is to attempt to build constructive working relationships with their local agencies as an initial strategy. This increases parents' moral authority if they have to use harder campaigning tactics at a later date.

2.   If a key individual becomes a real stumbling block – if they are simply 'uninspirable', or apparently incompetent or vindictive, remember that there is always a range of key people involved – an officer will report to a manager, or a local councillor, or a governor, so it is worth looking at how to get round a problem through engaging with different people.

> *LEAs vary a lot, but I take the view that even in the least good LEA, there must be someone who would like to change things. Don't be put off if you don't find one immediately.*

Winning people over

To create a change in attitudes you have to win people round.

> *At the end of the day, if you want things to change you are going to have to convince the people in office and in power to do things differently.*

The Audit Commission (2003, p.8) report looks at what distinguishes a 'good' authority from a 'bad' one. A key element is:

> *…interest and commitment at strategic leadership level.*

Parents can play a vital role in encouraging and supporting senior officers within local authorities to develop an interest in autism, and the commitment to building successful services. In doing this, building effective, respectful, working relationships is key.

Allies of all kinds are useful, for the information they bring, the links they can help you make, and to help develop interest in and concern for your cause.

> *To our surprise, at the public meeting the neuro-psychologist started arguing with the bosses that our concern over the low rate of diagnosis in our health authority was valid. I found out later that he had a child on the spectrum.*

> *It was wonderful finding [...], the educational psychologist. She made notes of all the things we're concerned about – statements, lack of autism awareness at the school, distress of core assessment, respite – she has given us a foot in the door, she has opened up a new channel of communication.*

Be open to finding unexpected allies. Don't assume that professionals don't want to help – they may be prevented from showing their support by the position they are in. Remember that circumstances change. The witness for the LEA at one parent's tribunal has become a key, long-term ally to one group of parents:

> We went to Tribunal because the provision my son was in couldn't meet his needs. The LEA called the head teacher of this school as a witness for their case against me. After the Tribunal, which we won, we got talking and I must have said how difficult it was to meet other parents. She offered to write to other parents and put us in touch with each other. That's how our group got started. She has been a terrific support in all kinds of ways; we still have the support group meetings at her school.

Be aware that you too may have attitudes that prevent you making progress. However evasive or formal officers seem, do not assume, for instance, that they do not care:

> The quickest way to alienate the professionals is to assume that they don't care. You cannot make progress if you believe that you are on the opposite side of a set of values. (Local authority officer)

You may find that you create room for change when you give up blaming particular individuals.

> There is a genuine feeling among some professionals that they could be doing their jobs better. They have an emotional investment in their work. If they are not blamed it's easier for them to accept that families are being let down, and that they can develop ways to do things better.

Some readers may find it helpful to look at this point at Chapter 7: 'Common dilemmas faced by parent campaigners' which illustrates different perspectives and approaches taken by a number of parent groups, and examines the consequences in one local authority of different groups of parents taking different approaches. Chapter 8 gives further background information on local government structures, people and processes.

Whom to approach, and when

> There's no formula for which path you should take or which doors to knock on – it is fluid. It took me a long time to work out that although the officers were the ones who dealt with policy, in our county council it

*was the elected councillors who had their hands on the purse strings,
and they were the ones who had to be persuaded to fund the new
approach.*

Parents need to find out who 'pulls the strings' locally when it comes to
deciding policy on key issues. Find out which officers are directly
responsible for the issue in hand, for example:

- officers in charge of SEN (e.g. the principal SEN officer) or
  the head of disabled children's social services team

- the director of education, or the director of children's services

In addition, there will be local individuals who are not directly responsible for services but who can be highly influential:

- parent partnership officers

- local councillors

- parent governor representatives.

We will discuss approaching all of these groups in this chapter. A full
account of how local authorities are structured, and the role of individuals within those structures, is contained in Chapter 8. Throughout, the
golden rule is that you should keep copies of any correspondence, dates
and notes of meetings and telephone calls, to build up a true record of
your efforts. This may be helpful if you need to show councillors or your
MP that you have made appropriate efforts to approach the authority.
See Chapter 6 for specific advice on approaching your MP.

How to find out who does what

Websites should give details of who does what within the relevant
department of your council or agency. You could ask to speak to the
council's information officer, or to the person who provides background
information on the council and its activities. If you cannot find out which
officer is dealing with the issue, you could write to the head of department or to the chief executive asking for your enquiry to be referred to
the appropriate department, and to be given the name of the individual
who will deal with it.

It is worth bearing in mind that even the people who work within
public authorities can find it very difficult to understand how they work,

and how to open 'closed' doors. The power balance in each local authority is different – so it is necessary to find out how yours works. Local democracy is often driven by personalities and can be very fluid: officers move jobs and councillors can be deselected or voted out of office.

Officers

These are people who are in paid positions within a council or local agency. It is normally most helpful for a group first to approach the officer or officers with responsibility for service development in their area, and then, or possibly in parallel, approach local councillors.

You can choose to take either a bottom-up or top-down approach to working with a particular agency. Some parents choose to escalate approaches up the officer 'food chain', writing to the director of the department that deals with their issue, and if that is unsuccessful, to the chief executive of the council or agency. One advantage of going steadily up the hierarchy in a systematic way is that you can demonstrate that you have operated appropriately, and that you haven't over-reacted by going straight for the 'big players'.

However, some people choose to go straight to the top and then to work backwards. A lot will depend on how sustainable and long-term a relationship you want to have: if this is what you are aiming for, it may make more sense to take things slowly and to ensure that you do not antagonise particular individuals by going over their heads unnecessarily. You may find that a junior officer will suggest you approach someone higher up in any case.

A first aim should simply be to get through the door and to interest officers in the potential for a constructive way forward. To this end, be aware that officers are often overwhelmed with work, and can easily feel swamped. Be constructive and offer a few pointers rather than a daunting shopping list of complaints and criticisms.

> Don't be surprised or put off by an initial rebuff – officers are under enormous pressure. [Y] wasn't put off when we rebuffed her initially. She rang back and said, 'I only want a little of your time', and then she came and did a very short presentation. She didn't say, 'So can I meet you next week?' She had good tactical understanding. (Local authority officer)

Some parents have found it so difficult to get meetings with senior managers that, when they do get through the door, they have treated the meeting as a rare one-off opportunity to raise all their concerns. But presenting the local authority with a long list of demands will simply leave officers focusing on how to get you out of their office.

Parent partnership officers

If you are working within education, you might want to contact your local parent partnership officer to discuss the issues, and perhaps for help in making contacts. Parent partnership officers can be valuable allies. The role of the parent partnership service is to empower parents. This means making parents better informed and more articulate about their needs, so that all parents and children are treated fairly and resources are fairly distributed.

> We had a brilliant parent partnership officer. She listened to us, plugged us in to places where our voice could be heard, came to meetings.

Parent partnership services should be neutral and independent of the LEA. Some are contracted out to the voluntary sector but most are based in the LEA's SEN department and usually they are funded by the LEA. Some parent partnership services are joint or triple funded by health and social services as well as the LEA.

Through parent partnership services, the LEA is responsible for:

- providing parents and schools with clear information about services and the range of options available

- including parental support groups and voluntary sector organisations in consultation on local policies for children with SEN

- informing all parents that all maintained schools are required to publish their SEN policies.

PACE is aware that parents' experiences of parent partnership officers are very mixed, depending on how genuinely independent their services are, and on the willingness of the individual officers to support parent campaigners. If working with the parent partnership officer is not fruitful in your authority, there will almost certainly be other champions who you can turn to. The key is to be persistent in tracking down your potential supporters. The Parent Partnership Network at CDC is a useful source of further information (see p.108 in the Resources section).

Councillors

Councillors are representatives of a particular local ward and a political party. Their work is voluntary, often additional to their paid 'day job'. As part of their role, they direct and oversee the work of the officers. As politicians, councillors may say that they have to balance the interests of different sections of the community – but it is always their unequivocal duty to represent the interests of the people in their ward. Many of the principles of approaching a councillor are therefore the same as for approaching an MP (see Chapter 6).

It can be very valuable for parents to approach local councillors personally, and in this situation it is often appropriate to raise your own personal case.

> Prior to the autism scrutiny we took a decision to tell people in difficulties to approach their county councillor. We helped them find out who their local councillor was, and suggested they go to the local surgery, or write and e-mail them and explain the problem. When it came to the scrutiny, lots of the councillors involved had already had contact with parents, and had heard about the problems at a personal level. I think that really made a difference.

A parent governor representative (see p.41 below) on one county council was instrumental in getting the council to investigate autism provision. Her motivation stemmed from seeing the problems first-hand.

> B. was climbing the walls. It was seeing how he was behaving, and what his mother was coping with, day in, day out, on her own, that did it for me. I felt that we had let her down. That really flagged up autism for me, and I didn't let it drop. (Parent governor representative)

Councillors are either members of the cabinet or of a scrutiny panel. Parents are likely to want to contact several councillors – their ward representative, the executive councillor or deputy for children's services, education or their particular area of concern, and the Chair of the appropriate scrutiny panel.

Before approaching councillors, parents may want to read recent council and the relevant scrutiny panel minutes in a particular area, to see which councillors are likely to be supportive or hostile. Parents can write to councillors at their home address, or care of the local authority. Keep letters short and clear. Most councillors will not know the background to the issue in the same way as officers, so brief them with the facts. Avoid jargon and acronyms. Try to get a relationship going, perhaps by inviting them to meet you and your child, or other parents with similar concerns. Be aware of their time constraints: councillors have a significant volume of council work, which they do over and above their 'day jobs'.

There is no rule about whether to approach councillors at the same time as officers, or only if efforts to work with officers are not successful.

> We had spent a long time trying to find someone at high level in the LEA who would listen to us. Finally we did – and he had power and influence. It was only then that we met with councillors, with his support.

You could try making links with individual executive councillors, and perhaps attending or requesting to give a submission to a relevant committee meeting on children's services. What you do not want to do is to 'wrong foot' the officers by a strident approach to councillors, so if you are approaching councillors early on in the process, do it constructively, and make sure you keep the officers in the loop.

Don't make assumptions about how much the councillor knows or doesn't know, or the extent of his or her influence. Some councillors are very committed and good at picking up on complex issues, and they may play an important role in discussions, but others are not as strong or as skilled. Many councillors struggle to understand the field of SEN and disability.

In some authorities councillors lack confidence and rely heavily on officers:

> We've tried approaching councillors. There was one whose heart was in the right place, her child was at my son's school, but they seem very weak and just refer us back to the principal education officer.

In other authorities the councillors have more power:

> I was struck by how much influence the councillors have, which was clear from the respect shown to them by the senior officer.

Parent governor representatives

Again in education, it also might be helpful to contact one of the parent governor representatives (PGRs) who are entitled to speak and vote on the committees and sub-committees dealing with education matters within the local education authority. PGRs are parent governors elected by other parent governors to provide a voice for all parents in their area in local decision-making. Some authorities have arrangements by which PGRs represent different locations within the authority, while in other authorities PGRs may represent distinct areas of education, including SEN. You may find individuals who are very determined.

> The parent governor representative took a really key role in moving things forward within the council. It turned out she had a child with SEN.

A parent governor representative told us that:

> The role of parent governor representatives is very powerful and under-utilised by parents. I've learned a lot about how to make the most of this role, and I'd like to be in touch with other parent governors who have taken on this role and want to be maximally effective.

Getting officers to engage with you

Is it ever possible to *force* officers to engage with your issues? Be aware that 'making a noise' doesn't mean that your message is going to be heard. It can leave you easier to manipulate: people will find ways to appear to be listening, but actually work out how to tiptoe round you.

One group of parents approached a local journalist who wrote an article about autism and how this group of parents had come together as a group. The day it was printed they telephoned and requested a meeting with the director of education. On being told that he was 'very busy', they told his secretary about the article. An hour later the secretary rang back with an appointment. The parents had been careful not to be confrontational in the article, but nevertheless the subsequent meetings did not have a good outcome. The parents felt that they were being played off between the director and officers using a 'good cop, bad cop' routine.

One way of establishing your interest and credentials with public authorities is to build on their efforts to consult users. Parents' experience of public authority consultation initiatives is the theme of the next chapter.

4. When the local authority approaches you

Public authorities are obliged to consult service-users on provision. Some parents have had a very positive experience of being approached by local agencies, and have found a way to capitalise on the proposals made to them.

> My paediatrician told me that services were all moving to a new building, and asked me to a public meeting about it. I asked two or three questions and afterwards the Chief Executive of the PCT [primary care trust] asked if I would be interested in being a user representative. He offered to pay us to run focus groups. We went back to him and said, 'We'll do a fantastic job for you, but we don't want payment: we want you to provide a room for us at the new centre.'

Consultations with parents work best when parents are involved in the design process, so that they are not just the objects of the consultation, but can also contribute to the process of developing it and carrying it out. Sometimes responding to consultations can lead to highly effective campaigns involving large numbers of people.

But parents also need to be aware of the danger of simply working to the authority's agenda, and should carefully assess what their group is getting from the relationship. If parents really are not getting anywhere, they need to be prepared to think again. And if they have succeeded in becoming a valued resource for the authority, parents will have some political capital that officers may be reluctant to squander.

Responding to public authority consultations
Once parents get known by the authorities, they may be inundated by requests to respond to consultations. While some are genuine and mean-

ingful efforts to engage with and understand the views of parents, others may be token efforts to fulfil a bureaucratic requirement to consult. Look for the real aim of the consultation, and work out if the intent is genuinely to bring about better outcomes for children and families.

> When they're going to consult, they usually send out an agenda and background papers. Make sure that you read them. If you feel that you will be genuinely listened to, go. If not, phone or e-mail your views so that you stay on their list, but don't waste your time.

For full information and invaluable advice about how to prepare, the CaF/CDC Parents Guide (2004) is a must – see References and key documents in the Resources section at the end of the Handbook. The guide provides very practical and specific pointers about organising your response.

Why respond to consultations?

Parents are often rightly cautious about contributing to tokenistic consultations, but some see benefits in responding. You don't need to respond passively to the agenda of the consultation; you can add your own points as well. It may, for instance, make sense to respond to a consultation on a respite centre because ultimately you want the agency to train up far more short break workers instead, or to go along to an inclusion forum because you want to see a new resource unit. A thoughtful response on one issue may help make sure that officers take you seriously on other issues. Another value in responding, and encouraging others to respond, is to let the agency know of the depth of feeling among parents.

> If they're asking open questions like, 'What do you want to see in future?' It's best to think about it in advance and touch base with other parents so that you go prepared with some constructive criticisms and constructive solutions. You might be able to come up with ideas that help them short-circuit months of work.

Show that parents expect transparency. If you suspect that major decisions have been made, for instance to close a particular school, and that consultations are 'window-dressing', ask what changes will be possible as a result of the consultation, and whether the report of the consultation will be made available to those who took part.

Sometimes parents can feel they are suffering from 'consultation fatigue', particularly when a group has been asked to consult its members in ways that do not really take parents' needs into account, or with insufficient time to do the work well. At the minimum in these cases, you can remind the authorities that they should reimburse parents who give up their time for child care and other costs.

Whenever there are problems, you can remind agencies that it is appropriate to expect any large-scale or controversial consultation to draw on genuinely independent expertise. This avoids problems that are often to do with a lack of experience or skill on the part of public authorities in designing and running consultations. There are important questions about the agenda behind the consultation, how it is to be carried out, and which target groups are to be involved.

What makes consultation meaningful – and what can we do if it isn't?

Some authorities have realised that working closely with parents has dramatically improved the services that they can provide, and these authorities have put significant resources into building genuine consensus with parents, rather than simply attempting to force them in particular directions. Other authorities have been perceived by parents as carrying out token consultation processes, simply to push through decisions that have effectively already been taken.

One authority has brought about a major reduction in statements through a sophisticated process of communication with parents. This involved sensitive letters to all parents concerned; a clear message that change would not take place without their and their school's agreement; and individual meetings with the parents of every child with a statement, with the option of having a lawyer or representative present if they wished. Only 44 out of 260 families chose to retain their child's statement. Since that time there has been a year-on-year reduction in statements, with just one of the original statements reinstated. No parent who gave up a statement has complained or appealed to SENDIST about this.

The officer who led the consultation believes that:

> It worked because the parents trusted us. The letter was not a fait accompli. If only 50% of parents had responded positively, or less, we would not have gone ahead.

Although parents did not play a major part in initiating this consultation, and there is considerable controversy around reducing statements (see Chapter 9, p.96), we have included it here because it is a genuine example of meaningful consultation. The same authority, in partnership with its two neighbours, has also taken part in a multi-agency, cross-authority review of provision for children with disabilities. Behind this was a key partnership: the project officer in charge – a senior social services manager – worked very closely with a parent of two children with autism. Parents were not the driving force in getting the review off the ground but it was an essential part of the review that parents and children with disabilities developed full ownership of it.

Parents were consulted at the outset on how they wanted to be involved. Many were cynical about the benefits of previous consultations. The review partners recognised the need to address parents' distrust and cynicism, and as a result a mechanism was set up to give parents a strategic overview of the process. This was a group of parents that would see all reports prior to publication and that had the power to call a wider group of parents to a meeting on any issue if they felt it necessary.

The parent who took an instrumental role in the process views the results very positively:

Every one of our recommendations has been addressed within the final report. The authorities had listened before, but this time parents felt genuinely heard. The professionals were thinking outside the box, and doing the inconceivable.

Parents continue to be at the heart of the process: four working groups, each co-chaired by a parent and a professional, have been set up to implement the review recommendations.

In other authorities parents have taken a more proactive, strategic role in consultations. A group of parents in north-east England have developed into a valued and trusted autism information resource for their local agencies, and often initiate research.

Two families were trying without success to access occupational therapy [OT] for their children. We met with the PCT to see if we could find a way forward. They asked us to produce information on the benefits of OT for children with autism and to research parents' views of the available provision. We did a literature search and found a few outcome studies in the USA and we did a comparative study of parents' views of provision and outcomes in two PCTs in our area. The results were conclusive. In the PCT where OT is established for children with autism, the comments were very positive, while the responses from the parents in the other PCT were more like hate mail. As a result OT is being established for children with autism in the PCT where it hasn't been available.

The painstaking work this group did to establish their legitimacy has paid off:

Our local authority wouldn't try to involve us in a consultation that wasn't serious, or a tick-box exercise. They know it wouldn't be productive. They respect and value us and they have an interest in preserving the relationship.

But many parents have experienced consultations to be token tick-box exercises. Even more worrying are consultations that parents perceive as window-dressing for controversial and unpopular decisions that have already been made.

Some parents have mobilised popular and political support for their concerns about such consultation processes. Plans to close excellent provision for children with special needs in one authority met very strong opposition within and beyond the borough. Some parents responded by refusing to stick to the narrow agenda of the consultation paper. Parents' concerns about the consultation process were voiced in a non-party political parliamentary debate devoted to the issue (secured by one of the constituency MPs).

The MP pointed to the lack of transparency in the consultation process about the real costs of the proposals, and the failure of the authority to seek a regional solution with other local authorities. Other parents campaigned through the local and national media, and a petition of 20,000 signatures was presented to the council, which was forced to drop its proposals.

What this shows is how vital it is for parents to engage in consultation processes, even if they suspect that the decision has already been taken. It is possible to force an authority to rethink and will also influence how they conduct consultations in the future. It can be highly effective to show that many parents (and potential voters) feel strongly about an issue.

Invitations to user groups and forums

Joining user groups is a very effective way for parents to learn how things work, who does what and who has influence. It is also an opportunity for professionals to get feedback from parents, and, if they are seeking parents' representatives to contribute at strategic level, to form a view of who they can work with.

Parents vary in their views of the effectiveness of such groups. Though they appreciate, for instance, that some multi-agency groups have a remit to bring together senior managers across institutional boundaries, they are frustrated when some individuals or agencies do not prioritise attending the meetings.

Some parents find that user groups can be frustrating and time-consuming, especially when there isn't a clearly defined, cohesive purpose. The danger is that these simply become a place for parents to 'off-load'.

> The LEA used to set up general 'parent–professional' meetings for us to raise issues. We used to hammer it in about autism. Actually they put themselves in quite a vulnerable position, it all got very personal. I felt quite sorry for them.

Some groups avoid this by having a level of formality. A pan-disability parents' advisory group in one county council is attended by representatives of all the parent groups and by senior officers in social care and education.

Some parents and local authorities are looking for more strategic ways to involve parents, for example in specific strategy groups rather than in a standing consultation forum. This may mean a smaller number of parents being involved, but taking a more influential role. This should not mean any less commitment from either the authority, or parents, to drawing on the breadth of parents' views, and it can lead to a more effective process. It would be important for the strategy group to have mechanisms for ensuring broad consultation with parents, for which the parent representatives might take or share responsibility. These could be written into the terms of reference for the group.

The CaF/CDC (2004) guidance provides a very useful list of questions (pp.24–26) for parents who have been asked to join a working group or committee.

Whether the initiative comes from you or from the authority, establishing your remit for working together is a vital step towards effective collaboration. The next chapter looks at this in more detail, along with some of the other issues involved in building constructive working relationships.

5. Building relationships and influence [1]

This section examines ways that parents can build their relationships and influence. This includes making meetings effective, identifying and then developing common ground, understanding the perspective of public authority decision-makers, and ensuring that you are successful in getting your message across. It also looks at how to assess your progress, and what you might do if you don't feel that you are making progress, including ways in which you might apply political pressure.

Building mutual respect

Collaboration must be based on behaviour that shows mutual respect. It is easy to fall into the trap of going to one extreme or the other – either being over-awed or over-critical. If you can find a way of respecting the professionalism of those you work with, you have more chance of getting them to respect you as a valuable resource, bringing first-hand knowledge about client groups and issues, and also to respect that you have a right for your views to be heard.

But some parents have felt that local authority officers have patronised them, or failed to recognise their efforts, time or commitment. Being undermined in this way is very damaging, and it is important to recognise it and to find ways to stop it happening.

I've heard of a very committed parent driving halfway across her county for a meeting that had been cancelled. All the professionals had been told but she had not. This kind of treatment is really

---

1   Throughout this chapter we refer to organisations and documents. Please see the Resources section at the end of the book for more information and how to contact and access these materials.

destructive. You must let them know that you're an equal, and ensure that you are treated with respect.

In your conversations and letters demonstrate an awareness of central government policy, new research and what other LEAs are doing. If you show that that you understand the current policy issues you will be less likely to be fobbed off.

Making meetings work

Meetings take different forms – from a one-off visit to see one or two individuals on a particular topic, to those that are much larger, possibly on a regular basis, involving a Chair, formal agendas and minutes. Preparation is vital to a meeting's success. You need to develop an idea of what might be realistic and achievable outcomes from a meeting, but don't try to achieve too much: some parents propose a maximum of three aims per meeting, while others stick to just one.

The CaF/CDC (2004) guidance has very useful pointers for preparation for conduct during, and follow-up after meetings, and a checklist to help you understand and fully participate in more formal committees and working groups (p.21).

If parents have initiated the meeting, they can offer to send a draft agenda beforehand, and give officers time to look into the issues and find the information they need. Don't 'drop them in it': give participants time to find answers to your questions.

Accurate minutes are very important, particularly when a meeting is covering an issue where there is conflict or controversy. Be sure in advance of the meeting that the minute-taker will record all decisions accurately, and check the minutes when they are circulated, which should be as a draft for approval. Where it isn't a formal meeting with minutes, it can be helpful to write a note to thank the people concerned, and in doing so highlighting any actions that they might have agreed to or points of principle that they acknowledged.

Clarify the time available for the meeting. At the end, always make sure there's an agreed action plan, however brief, and, if you want one, a follow-up meeting arranged – in fact, because change is likely to be a long-term process, getting another meeting might be one of your three objectives.

Don't waffle. There can be many distractions in a meeting, and temptations to go off at a tangent. Always try to remember what the meeting is for. Be business-like and stick to the main matter in hand.

We've got a system where I tap my parent colleague on the arm to let her know that she's going off at a tangent – and she'll do the same to me.

It is the task of the Chair to rise above the issues and find the neutrality to steer the process forwards as well as to chase progress between meetings and check minutes for accuracy. If you feel that the Chair is not pulling the meeting together, you can ask questions to move things along, for example 'Could I just clarify what decision we made there?' or 'I don't understand how what x has just said relates to the matter on the agenda'.

Experienced parent campaigners are adept at finding tactful ways to move discussion forward.

I'm very succinct and I say what I think, but I try to say it in a positive and productive manner. When I think they're on the wrong foot I say things like, 'Could we look at it this way?' or 'I'm not sure that we're quite getting things right.'

Be sensitive in how you seek information. Officers can easily react defensively to questions and demands. Don't spring questions on professionals – they often won't know the answers and they won't appreciate being put on the spot. Everything rests on how you say it.

I asked, 'How are these decisions made? Who knows about autism?' They were defensive. I suppose I was attacking them.

Parents may talk of feeling intimidated by professionals but it may help them to understand that professionals are often even more scared of having to face awkward questions, and that they will appear uninvolved, act evasively or retreat into 'bureaucratic working' because they are frightened. (Local authority officer)

But asking simple questions can help officers to make sense of the issue. When you seek information, what is very important is the intent behind your questions. If you are understood to be genuinely committed to taking things forward with the authority, such questions will not be perceived as threatening. You can help everyone if you ask for clarification.

Being a parent you can say, 'Could you translate that, please, into language I can understand?'.

Officers should be able to communicate with parents without using jargon, so it is quite appropriate to ask them to explain it. If you don't have the confidence to ask at the time, make a note of the phrase and ask someone privately later.

I used to get very confused by people saying things like 'There is some quality protects money,' which sounds like ungrammatical rubbish until I found out that there is a government scheme called 'Quality Protects' which gave grants for certain projects. Don't let jargon put you off – you pick it up more easily than you think you're going to. Most of us had never heard of SEN, EPs [educational psychologists], ASDs at one time, and I bet we all know what they are now.

How you share information is also important. If you show that you value transparency but respect confidentiality, you will develop officers' respect.

Officers have to feel confident that they can trust you, and that nothing that they tell you will disadvantage them.

It is also important that you are rigorous and fair in collecting information.

You need to let people have the sources for your information: 'We've had 600 calls on our helpline… 40 parents came to this meeting…'

Issues of confidentiality, ethics and data protection are important.

We give each new member a sheet with an opt-out clause so that we don't contact parents who do not want to be contacted to contribute their views.

Identifying and developing common ground

It is important to seek common ground with officers. If all parties feel that they are serious about what they are doing, and that they genuinely share common ground, the process is likely to go well.

It's very important to understand whether officers see your concern as their problem. If they don't, consider how you can communicate this effectively. Develop an informed picture, drawing on different sources – the views of a range of parents and professionals. Once you have the agreement of professionals that you have a common understanding, you can begin to work on a common problem. (Local authority officer)

Whether it is the causes of autism or the merits of different educational interventions, autism is an area that attracts different – and strongly held – views. If you demonstrate your awareness that such differences exist you will show that you are knowledgeable and not naive. There is a level of skill involved in presenting and acknowledging different views. Parents who can do this will have far more impact, even if they eventually come down in a well-argued way on one side. Equally, highlighting differences can be a useful process for digging deeper and identifying the common ground that does exist, which may be where most change can be made.

Parents will be much more effective if they understand the perspective of local authority officers. For instance, special educational needs is generally acknowledged as the most pressurised area of work in education. There are huge competing demands, which are very hard to manage and predict, and parents who are fighting for one of the most important issues of their lives. Officers may not be able to be up-front about some of their problems. They are balancing their attempts to support services that are under pressure with the needs of children with disabilities which are becoming more complex and for which there is inadequate provision.

It will help enormously if you understand the tensions that local authority officers are up against, and if you understand that the bureaucracy and pace of change gets us down as much as it does you. (Local authority officer)

Most importantly, try to show an understanding that the nature of many problems is to a large extent structural, rather than personal:

What we valued in working with [two parents] was their understanding that the issues we struggle with are systemic. They would frequently remind us that they knew that there needed to be initiatives at national level for the problems to be solved. If you say, 'That's all very well, but we can't wait', you simply alienate the professionals you are seeking to work with. (Local authority officer)

I think it helped that we were willing to say 'This must be a problem for you statutory agencies, what can we do to ease things a bit now, and what can we discuss as a long-term need that we have to work towards more slowly than we'd all like?', rather than 'The whole system stinks, it's all hopeless'. I often believed the latter, but also presumed that the officers themselves felt like that in their heart of hearts, but had to get on and do the job within considerable constraints.

One of the advantages of this approach is that you may be able to elicit a joint approach to a national body, for example the DfES or the Local Government Association. It is still very unusual for parents and local authorities jointly to highlight the pressures in the system, but when they do, the message can be very powerful. Effectively it is saying 'We recognise that local disputes between parents and authorities are symptoms of system failures higher up and we want national bodies to do something about it.'

Putting across your perspective

Making an effective case as a parent campaigner involves a combination of knowing the issues and arguments around autism, and the particular area or problem you are meeting to discuss, and communicating clearly and persuasively.

Making an effective case: your arguments

Parents who are able to use reasoned arguments and hard facts and figures on top of highlighting the 'rightness' of their case are most likely to achieve results.

If you are seeking strategic change, the first step is to ensure that there is awareness of the need that the authority faces, now and in the future. It is very hard to move forward unless all agencies appreciate that there has been an increase in the recognised number of children with a diagnosis of autism. One county council was still reporting to members in 2002 that the prevalence rate for autism was 5 per 10,000, when the Medical Research Council figure of the previous year stated 60 per 10,000 (Medical Research Council 2001). If you find out the total number of children in your authority through the government's statistics website, you can use the MRC prevalence rate to work out how many children are likely to have autism:

$$\frac{\text{Total number of children in your authority} \times 60}{10,000} = \text{Likely number of children with autism}$$

For example: from the Census 2001 website (see the Resources section under 'Other resources' for details of how to use this site), we know that in 2001 there were 23,886 children under 19 in Hartlepool. This means that the likely number of children with autism was 143.

- *Warning 1.* The Census 2001 site only breaks down population by local authority. This will give you the right numbers in relation to your council and LEA, but if you are talking to another body such as your primary care trust, you will need to check if their boundaries are different.

- *Warning 2.* Very few parliamentary constituencies have the same boundaries as local authorities. You may be able to work out roughly how many of your MP's constituents have children with autism using the local authority data – for instance, some local authorities have two parliamentary constituencies. Alternatively, you can offer an average likely figure as follows: given that the average MP has 67,000 constituents, the average likely number of children with autism in each constituency will be 402.

You may also find it helpful to demonstrate an understanding of the policy context referred to in Chapters 9 and 10, to explain in a 'no-blame' way the struggle that public agencies have in meeting the needs of children with autism. Additionally, here are some key references you may find useful in stating your case:

- There are at least 90,000 children with autism in the UK, but only 7,500 specialist educational places (Jones 2002).

- 72 per cent of schools are dissatisfied with the extent of their teachers' training in autism (Barnard *et al.* 2002).

- Only 20 per cent of teachers who have a pupil with autism will have had any training in autism, and the training they have had is usually half a day or less (Barnard *et al.* 2002).

- One in five children with autism are excluded from school at some point (Barnard *et al.* 2000).

- In the past ten years, there has been a 600 per cent increase in SEN and Disability Tribunal hearings concerning children with autism, showing the growing conflict between parents and LEAs over school provision. Autism is the highest single disability category of SENDIST cases. (See SENDIST annual reports for further information, available from www. sendist.gov.uk and see also p.108 in the Resources section.)

It is helpful to draw on established and dispassionate sources to support your case, such as the DfES/DH *Autistic Spectrum Disorders Good Practice Guidance* (Department for Education and Skills/Department of Health 2002), and to offer encouragement rather than blame if you know things are being done well elsewhere. The online examples of the Guidance can be very useful here. (See Resources section, p.106, for the web details.)

At a conference on SEN and education law, officers listening to presentations on the problems facing families were heard to say, 'I feel completely destroyed', 'I feel like I've been bashed round the head' and 'I'm going to leave completely drained.' So, whenever possible, try to have solutions in mind to the problems you are identifying. Be clear precisely what you're asking for and come up with ideas to solve the problems involved. We are at our most effective when we can inspire and enthuse people to work for change.

Making an effective case: presentation skills

The facts about autism and lack of provision are persuasive of themselves, but it can take time to develop the skills to put the message across.

> I've gradually built up confidence doing presentations on autism to foster carers, child-minders and GPs, and I'm now working with educational psychologists... I've been asked to do a presentation for the local authority strategy group – the people who apparently have 'the vision and the money'!

It pays dividends to think in advance about how to present your case. Learn as much as you can about the audience – where are they coming from? What can you connect with in them? What will make them more likely to take an interest in your issues? If you are making a presentation to councillors, how might your ideas help them win new voters? What angle will appeal to them?

Parents continually stress the importance of communicating professionally:

> It's hard to be succinct, keep your temper and be patient, but it's essential. It works.

It is important to give evidence for arguments, but be aware of the dangers of presenting dry figures and bad news. Look for ways to demonstrate that the changes in provision you seek will have positive results for both children with autism and their families.

Think carefully about possible ways to inspire your audience. Try always to present possible, realistic solutions, as well as outlining the problems. Spell out the benefits for the children, not just for the parents, and also for the professionals. Think carefully about how to get the reality of autism across, and the evidence of benefits.

While officers may know a great deal about educational theory, remember that councillors may not know much about education, and less still about autism. They may find it hard to take in the finer points of your argument.

> Councillors aren't specialists, and if you don't live with autism, the issues are really complicated and hard to understand. It was no good bombarding the councillors with the scientific research – we had to give them the information in bite-sized chunks. But the officer had been an educational psychologist and he really understood the issues.

There can be advantages to councillors not being specialists:

> The professional managers are often so mired in the issues of different budget streams that they don't see the potential savings that can come from thinking differently. But local councillors see the logic more easily. 'Do you realise that if you give me £3,000 more per head you won't have to pay £100,000 on x or y?' Figures mean something to councillors, they aren't so bureaucratic. They are more likely to identify with us as parents, and they also are aware that we are voters.

Telling personal stories can be a good way to communicate the problems, as long as you are doing it to illustrate a wider point, not to try to get your own individual child's needs met, or to meet your own need to have your personal experience listened to.

> There's a place for your emotional experience, but keep it within reins. I heard councillors gasp when a parent explained that her 11-year-old had never been out of the house without adult supervision. It also made an impression on them when another parent explained that her child had a 2:1 in astrophysics but can't make tea on his own. And they began to realise that it is possible to help these kids, when she explained how the university had supported him.

Parents find that once they have developed a relationship and shown that they understand officers' points of view they can talk quite directly, as long as they make their points calmly and without blame. And once they have earned respect they can, if they are thoughtful about it, speak from the heart:

> I told one committee, 'It's not your fault, but you don't think about respite like a parent. It's not respite if the parent's not happy about where their child is. It's no good having just one option for everyone.'

Over time, and having developed experience, some parents feel able to take more risks. One parent, a professional disability consultant with many years' experience in policy forums, feels that she can be impassionate, and say 'outrageous things'. She often prefaces these by saying that she is 'in parent mode':

> I'm prepared to get into conflict. I say things like 'I'm sorry, but parents don't like that', or, 'But you said that ten years ago, and a generation of children has gone through and nothing has changed'. Sometimes I use humour, and I know how to move people. But I'm professional – I know my stuff. I have a reputation for knowing about autism and I normally have something to say about the bigger picture. And I never talk about my own child's needs.

Some parents are skilled in using humour:

> The professionals survive by using really black humour. I've found that if I can tap into it I can really make a link with them.

> I heard a parent give a talk on 'managing challenging behaviour'. She was talking about the challenging behaviour of the professionals. She described how parents have to cope with a triad of impairments: health, education and social services, and gave some excellent examples of what the challenging behaviour of professionals can lead to.

Assessing progress – and what to do if things don't seem to be moving forward

It can be very difficult to chart progress. You may think that you are not achieving anything, when in fact you may be having substantial impact. You do not know, for instance, when you write to make a case for something to a local authority policy officer, whether others have made the same case as you – your letter may be decisive in reinforcing an argument made by others, but you may not even get a reply. And when things do change, it's often difficult to know precisely what led to the change, and how much it's down to your efforts.

It's also the case that achieving change is a long-term process and sometimes parents have to make difficult decisions about when they should take issue on a question and when to let something rest. Sometimes, though not always, the long-term relationship is more important than succeeding with a particular outcome.

It may help you assess progress if, at the outset, you work out what it might look like. What would be realistic and achievable goals to aim for? Many parents emphasise that it is no small achievement to create an environment where genuine dialogue can take place with decision-makers, and once this is achieved, it should be possible to develop goals jointly with the professionals.

When progress happens, it can mean a lot to the officers and councillors that parents appreciate the efforts they have made:

> When my local authority opened middle-school provision for children with autism in mainstream schools I wrote to thank the director. The Ofsted report had been quite negative about them not providing 'value for money', and I wanted them to know that I thought they provided huge value. Later I discovered that the director had told many other people about the letter I'd written.

But sometimes there doesn't seem to be progress. Sometimes parents' efforts to build relationships over time are not productive. Some parents report that meetings take place but don't seem to lead anywhere. Other parents feel skilfully manipulated into an appearance of dialogue. If things are not working, it may be helpful to seek ways to apply political pressure within the authority.

Making use of political processes in local authorities

There are various ways that parents and groups might seek to apply political pressure. The following sections draw on information covered in Chapter 8.

Is there a dissenting faction within the controlling political group on your council? They may be prepared to put pressure on the leadership to think again. Or you might find it possible to target councillors from the controlling group who represent marginal wards: few councillors will want to defend a policy openly that might lose them their seat at the next local election. You might want to weigh up the risks of taking your argument to opposition councillors and proposing that they take it up as a political campaign. You should, however, be careful to ensure that this is carried out in the spirit of a policy information exercise which you have taken to all parties, rather than a party-political manoeuvre.

Councillors can also be very vulnerable to deselection by their political parties. Very few people are involved in local politics so at ward level often only six to ten people could deselect a councillor through joining that councillor's political party and taking an active part in ward meetings. However, remember that taking an active part in ward meetings is in itself no small piece of work. It can take a lot of time and energy and divert you from the key focus of autism services for children. We would advise that you only use this approach if (a) you're very confident of achieving your ends and/or (b) you genuinely enjoy the whole process of local politics, at a level that is broader than the single issue of children's services and autism.

Parents who use political means to achieve their goals in this way run the risk of damaging their reputation. And it is important not to use such tactics during election campaigns as you may be committing a criminal offence under the Representation of the People Act 1983. If a parent group is constituted as a charity, then the Charity Commission guidelines on political campaigning will also apply – and these need to be followed if you want to retain your charitable status.

It is possible that opposition councillors might take up your cause as a segment of a wider campaign to score political points against the majority party. This can assist the 'noise' around your case, but remember that it may be very counter-productive in that it may alienate those who actually have power. If, however, it is a particularly sensitive issue, getting opposition support for your case can at least raise awareness and make it more of a priority.

Petitions and deputations

Petitions and deputations are both forms of representation that you should consider. Petitions can be very significant in a crisis. In one local authority parents and teachers collected 20,000 signatures in a campaign against the closure of several special schools. The council was forced to back down.

Procedures governing the presentation of petitions vary and are usually included in a council's standing orders – the rules that govern council proceedings. These should be consulted before you organise any kind of representation.

Deputations involve a group of people making a special case. Apart from at scrutiny panels, shortage of time means that councils rarely permit an outside group to represent their members' case, but if you do get the chance it can be a good opportunity to put across your view and deal with questions.

Write to the chief executive to ask whether the council will consider receiving a deputation – the chance for a number of individuals representing your group or a number of groups to put their case. Outline the issue and the number of people affected. But remember that a deputation is only as persuasive as the voices of the people involved.

If these methods are not successful, you may want to think about how you can draw on external levers to influence things, described in the next chapter.

6. Using external levers of influence [1]

MPs, the media and the law

If parents want to make change happen, they have to engage with officers, and where appropriate local councillors, using the strategies set out in the previous chapter. But officers and councillors will also be subject to two types of external influences. First, MPs and local media can force an issue higher up their agenda. Some parents have had a major impact when contacting their MP, particularly when direct approaches to local agencies have not achieved results. Second, autism may also be higher on the agenda when the authority is involved in a legal case. Winning a SENDIST tribunal provides parents with an opportunity to make a wider point beyond the individual child in question and potentially to bring about general improvements in policy and provision.

Contacting your MP

Some parents and groups have found it useful to contact their MP, either to help them lobby their local authority for general improvements in services or about their own particular cases.

Many MPs have become powerful advocates for children with autism, supporting autism initiatives in parliament and raising their concerns within parliament and with ministers, because of the impact on them of hearing their constituents' experience. Dr Stephen Ladyman MP

---

[1]   In this chapter we make several references to resources and organisations which are detailed more fully in the Resources section at the end of the Handbook.

says that it was the persistence of mothers of children with autism in his constituency surgeries that sparked his interest in autism. He went on to become the founding chair of the All-Party Parliamentary Group on Autism and became the first health minister to have autism as a specific responsibility.

In one campaign, parents so successfully lobbied their MP that he secured a debate in parliament, and this contributed to a reversal of a local authority proposal (see p.47).

Technically MPs can help only with matters for which parliament or central government is responsible, i.e.:

> Matters such as school closures and grants which are dealt with by the Department for Education and Skills (but not day to day problems involving schools which are run by their governors and your local education authority). (House of Commons Information Office 2003, p.3)

However, almost all MPs do significant amounts of constituency work, even in areas where the local authority has direct responsibility. Although they have no formal influence in such areas, MPs are sometimes prepared to act as advocates for individual parents and parents' groups in their dealings with local authorities, and may be successful where doors are closed, or where parents have had a poor response to their concerns. As long as you have genuinely tried to work with your local authority before approaching your MP, your concerns are unlikely to be dismissed. A former parliamentary assistant to a Labour MP says:

> Don't think that the issue is too small, a large majority of MPs' postbags is about potholes, litter and grass verges – on the up side this does make the bigger issues stand out.

Making the most of your MP

If the council is run by a different political party to that of your MP, this might affect how your MP can be most effective as a local advocate. In this case, it might be better for the MP to write to the director of the relevant department, rather than the lead cabinet member. An MP from a different party might be more willing to be publicly critical of the council, if you have decided to request their help in seeking press coverage.

You could look up your MP on a political website like www.epolitix. com. If he or she is a government MP, perhaps even a minister or a parliamentary private secretary (120 MPs are members of the government), then criticising government policy is unlikely to go down well – but that approach might well work with an opposition MP. If they are connected to the government, you might be more successful if you focus on the fact that 'their' local authority is not yet properly implementing government policy.

Initial contact

Rather than writing to request a formal meeting, the best route to an MP is for one or two parents to go to the MP's surgery to explain the issues briefly and ask for the MP's assistance. Some surgeries are drop-in, others by appointment. Constituency offices are in the telephone directory, or you can call the parliament switchboard (020 7219 3000) and ask for the parliamentary office of your MP, which should know when the next surgery is.

You should take with you a concise written summary of your concerns – enough for an MP's assistant who was not at the surgery to pick up the file later and understand the problem. You should bring along copies of previous correspondence, evidence of efforts to engage with the local authority, minutes of any meetings, etc. These should demonstrate that you have made genuine efforts to work with your authority. MPs will assume that you are there to talk about an individual case, but you can also ask for support in relation to a wider campaign. Either way, you will need to explain carefully what it is that you want, but are not getting, from local public agencies.

In the first instance, generally asking for advice and support is probably the best approach, as it allows the MP to take some ownership of the situation. A good initial outcome is if he or she proposes writing to key local players, to ask for information about the issue.

> I think it's a bit like seeing a doctor. It's important that they take charge of dealing with the problem. But if there is a step that you think would be particularly helpful, like requesting a meeting with the authority, you could say that there is something that you think might help.

MPs may also help in attracting local media coverage (see below). If the MP seems receptive to your issue, you could invite him or her to attend part of a parents' group meeting. It is worth emphasising the number of children (and their parent voters) affected by autism, as this is likely to motivate an MP to get involved. (Chapter 5 contains tips on how you can calculate the number of children with autism in your constituency.)

It is important to remember that MPs are not obliged to help you with local matters, and that they vary hugely in their commitment to their constituencies. There is no formal procedure for complaining about your MP if he or she fails to help you. Unless the MP is corrupt or has committed a criminal offence, the only remedy is for his or her constituency party to deselect him or her before the next election – or failing that, for the electorate to vote for someone else.

A note of caution…

Some parents have found their MPs' efforts unhelpful. One parent did not know what to make of a letter sent to the MP by the director of education, which the MP had copied to her without a covering letter:

> The letter said that I 'was a great disappointment, very unreasonable'. Had the director's view of me convinced the MP not to have any more to do with our concerns?

Using the media

The media is a very powerful influence, and there are some important cases of it making all the difference. Local media have played a key role in parents' campaigns to defend services against closure or cuts, for instance, and national media attention may have played a significant role in keeping autism on the government agenda in recent years. But we have found little evidence that using local media benefits the development of effective relationships with service-providers, and we cannot stress strongly enough how often it can be counter-productive. The local press may be helpful in bringing about an initial engagement with public authorities, but there are clear dangers in 'bouncing' professionals into meeting you. If you are thinking about using the media, always be clear in your mind why you are doing it, and think long and hard about the possible dangers. This is not to say that we categorically advise against using the media, but rather to emphasise how important we feel it is that parents are clear why they are publicising their issues. It is dangerous to assume it will automatically help.

Some parents are very wary of involving the local media, even when they feel that they are not making progress and have nothing to lose. They caution that parents have no control over what is printed or broadcast, and stress that local papers may have their own axe to grind, with the local council, for instance, and may be inaccurate or overly sensationalist:

> They said things that weren't true, and they ignored half of what I'd said.

Even if there is careful attention to facts, and parents get the press coverage they seek, the impact may only be beneficial short-term.

> In Autism Awareness Week one of the mothers organised a nice double-page spread about our group in the local paper. It wasn't antagonistic to the authority, but it talked about the hardships and difficulties. We planned it beforehand, decided that we would not be drawn into anything political. It was good, because it wasn't confrontational, but it did show that we weren't going to disappear.

However, although the media coverage helped these parents to get through the doors of the director of education, the subsequent meetings did not go well. It seems that the department felt manipulated into meeting the parents, and consequently looked for ways to out-manoeuvre them.

MPs have their own electoral interests in getting local media coverage of their efforts; they are likely to want to be seen as 'hot' on community issues. They may be interested in seeking media attention, and may bring about helpful media coverage.

An MP raised concerns aired by local parents about poor autism services to the local authority, proposing that they study good practice in a neighbouring authority, which she also contacted. Simultaneously she released the letter to the local press. This may have been an effective way of embarrassing the local authority while keeping the individual parents out of the limelight. The local authority concerned had little option but to make contact with the neighbouring authority and draw on their experience.

One campaigning group has decided to work almost entirely in the public eye, to develop better health services for children and adults with autism.

> Things are really bad here, we have very low rates of diagnosis – it's only since we've started campaigning that they've even employed someone who is able to diagnose children under five, and over-five-year-olds are still sent out of the county to be diagnosed. It's a real black hole.

The group had several meetings with their local health authority to air concerns about low rates of diagnosis, but the meetings did not lead to a concrete outcome. The group then decided to tackle the problem in public, with the sustained help of a local journalist and the local MP. The lead campaigner, an adult with Asperger syndrome, wrote several articles about his concerns for the local paper. After one article the local journalist approached the health authority and gained their agreement to try to work with the group. The lead campaigner responded to the news of this agreement through the newspaper.

> I wrote 'Let's make it a big public meeting.' Of course they couldn't back down. About 75 professionals came, from all the different agencies, and another 75 parents. We had all the people from the authorities on the stage and there were a lot of angry and frustrated parents; some of them were in tears. I held on to the microphone – I didn't want the really angry speakers to get hold of it. We asked the professionals a lot of questions and gave them a deadline to come back with answers.

The authority's joint commissioning unit has responded to the deadline by setting up a working group involving parents and other autism campaigners to deliver improvements, which will shortly meet for the first time. This is clearly an achievement, and the group feels that there is a promising energy among the professionals involved. But the campaigners also recognise that progress made by the working group will be the real test of their effectiveness, and that it is too early to judge this.

Some parents have used the press to draw attention to their individual plight, and some have witnessed benefits for their particular families. Desperate to get what she considered the necessary provision for her daughter with autism, one mother decided to go on hunger strike, and with her husband contacted their local paper about their case. The national press, TV and radio picked up their story, and Iain Duncan-Smith, then Conservative leader, and the opposition spokesperson for SEN both met the parents. Shortly afterwards the LEA offered the family a much better support package for their daughter.

> The fact that we attacked the LEA in a robust manner and got the publicity basically forced them to increase our daughter's support. We had articles produced and reporters harassing the LEA every time they were about to have a meeting to discuss her... My answer is go public, get support and harass the LEA into submission.

This kind of coverage is unlikely to make the council change policy, even if it benefits the individual parents. But it can perhaps create a head of steam that makes a department more motivated to reach policy solutions with other groups of parents.

> It's sometimes helpful for LEA officers to have a pressure point. They also feel that there is a lack of provision, and it helps them to make the case internally. (Local authority officer)

One mother whose child with Asperger syndrome had been excluded from his mainstream school, and who was receiving very little educational support, found herself telling a local journalist about her son's problems at an unrelated event. To her shock the local newspaper ran the story with a sensational headline. The parent concerned did not feel that it was helpful, and officers and councillors who were already meeting with parents to try to make changes maintain that it did not influence them.

This parent also wrote a leaflet to hand out to people who asked her why her child was out of school, asking those concerned to write on her son's behalf to the government minister for SEN.

Parents emphasise the benefits of building a relationship with a journalist who can be trusted, but it is important to understand that journalists themselves do not have editorial control over what they write, and that fair coverage could take on a different slant in the final version.

If you do decide to seek media attention, the following tips may be helpful.

Local or national?

Remember that however big a story you think you have, the national press will feel they've heard it all before. It is likely to be the exception rather than the rule that they will take an interest in your case, and unless you have an existing 'in' with journalists, it may not be worth your effort to go down the national route. However, they may pick up an interesting story if it is already in the public domain at a local level.

Making contact

If you decide to cold-call your local newspaper, ask for the education (or children's issues) section or the news desk. Write out the main points beforehand and make it as brief as possible. Relate your story to a recent national news item or a recent piece of research if you can. Journalists are keen on human-interest stories, which means drawing on your own personal situation. Be aware that you may find this invasive, and decide in advance what aspects of your personal story you are prepared to talk about.

If the journalist seems interested, always keep a record of their name and number, and periodically keep them informed of developments (but not so often that they get tired of hearing from you!).

Writing letters, or your own article

Letters in response to an article help keep an issue in the public eye. Even if you haven't been the subject of the original story, you can capitalise on it by adding your own experience or opinion. Bear in mind that:

- letters speaking on behalf of or signed by several people or groups may have an extra chance of being published

- the shorter the letter, the greater its chances of being published. You should try and make just one point, even if there are hundreds of points you are desperate to get over

- it's good to be pithy and, if at all possible, humorous.

The best way to keep control over content is to offer to write a personal piece for a local newspaper. Some newspapers have a format that enables readers to do this. But you do need to be able to write in a style that will suit the paper. If you contact your local paper to suggest this, they are likely to want to see your piece before committing themselves.

Using the law

There are a number of legal means that parents can have recourse to, but, quite apart from being costly and stressful, there are very limited in what they can achieve in terms of altering an agency's policy. While parents may have to use judicial remedies for their own children, PACE does not advise parents to use them as the primary levers to change policy more broadly, unless a test case is the only way to demonstrate to the local authority that they are acting unlawfully in their interpretation of government policy.

Sadly many parents find that they have to go to SENDIST to get the educational provision that their child needs. SENDIST decisions apply only to the individual cases that they refer to. A smaller number of parents will bring a judicial review against an LEA or another local agency. Judicial reviews are a form of court proceeding in which a judge reviews the lawfulness of a decision made or action taken by a public body. They are a challenge to the way in which a decision has been made. Judicial reviews do set precedents in case law, but these precedents can only be accessed through further legal proceedings; they don't force the LEA to change policy – they just make it more likely that a later legal challenge would be successful.

There is no automatic mechanism that allows parents who win a tribunal appeal or bring a successful judicial review to translate this into better provision for children in the authority more generally. However, there are some things you can do to try to alter the agency's policy after your case:

- Point out to the relevant officers that it would be cheaper in the long run to change policy than lose a succession of cases. However, you should bear in mind that the agency may not lose a future case even if it appears very similar to your own unless the facts are exactly the same.

- Make it clear that you will use your experience to support other parents who have similar difficulties, thus increasing the likelihood of other cases coming forward.

- Threaten to go to the media with a story along the lines that 'My LEA/primary care trust made my family go through the hell of a long legal process. They lost and even now they are denying support to other children in a similar position.'

Obviously, all of the above require you to have significant mental strength and other resources. Many parents feel that it is really better to try to mend bridges with local agencies after tribunal and court cases, and that continuing to fight may actually be less effective for other families than supporting efforts to build dialogue with the authority.

Local authority complaints procedures

If you are unhappy with the way you have been treated in your individual case by your local authority, you can access the local authority complaints procedure in your council. Contact the council's information officer or see their website for more information – you cannot go to the local government ombudsman (see below) without first having tried your council's own complaints procedure.

Contacting the ombudsman

Contacting the local government ombudsman (LGO) may be an effective way of holding your local authority to account. The equivalent body for the NHS is the health service ombudsman. Local authorities are expected to act reasonably promptly, to treat local people fairly and to fulfil their legal duties. You can go to the LGO if your complaint is about maladministration, i.e. an organisation failing to follow its own procedures or taking too long to do something, or not doing something it had agreed to do (e.g. failing to provide for a child's needs as set out in his or her statement).

> This is a useful and fairly straightforward means of action, which has a number of advantages. It's a DIY operation, which costs nothing. The ombudsman reacts quickly, usually within 29 days, and if he judges that an investigation is called for it begins immediately. Local authorities have to take notice of him whether they want to or not.

Most cases brought to the LGO are directed at individual redress, although they can result in requirements to councils to put right administration procedures. In a large number of cases councils accept in the course of an investigation that they have done something wrong and offer to put it right. This initiative may come from the council itself or, more often, be proposed by the ombudsman's office. If the ombudsman is satisfied with the remedial action offered by a council, he or she will regard the complaint as 'locally settled' and discontinue the investigation.

The local media may report LGO decisions or concerns, and the council's response, for instance, if the LGO finds that a council is struggling to meet its statutory obligations. To find out more about how to approach the local government ombudsman, see its website at www.lgo.org.uk and see the Resources section, p.108.

Using administrative procedures to hold authorities to account

Building effective partnerships of trust and respect between local public authorities and parents is extremely difficult where authorities have taken what appear to be entrenched positions and large numbers of parents have had to resort to legal routes to meet their children's needs.

However, some parents are exploring the possibility of drawing on their experience at SENDIST to influence local authority decision-making. One parent who has successfully fought a SENDIST case is attempting to use the local authority complaints procedure and other mechanisms to challenge what he and other parents perceive to be a tacit policy on the part of the LEA to oppose a particular early intervention programme, and the flawed basis on which the local authority attempts to defend its decisions at Tribunal. In this way he hopes to force reform of the SEN decision-making practice within the authority.

The parent drew on his rights under the Data Protection Act and the Freedom of Information Act to look at the authority's file on his case, and discovered that an important e-mail giving cautious support to his preferred choice of provision had been removed. He believes that if the local authority can be demonstrated to be guilty of maladministration and to have opposed his chosen form of intervention on flawed evidence, the outlook will be better for other children in the borough. He contacted his MP and asked him to put pressure on officers and council-lors to review SEN decision-making, and to look at the resources put into fighting Tribunals. His MP has suggested that he use the complaints procedure, and contact in turn the SEN department manager, the director of education and then the local government ombudsman. If the ombudsman rules in his favour the MP has offered to take up the ruling with the chief executive.

The mechanisms described in this chapter all have their place when warranted by the circumstances. However, parents may differ in their analysis of circumstances and the decisions they make about what approach to take and when. The next chapter looks at some of the issues involved in taking different approaches to campaigning.

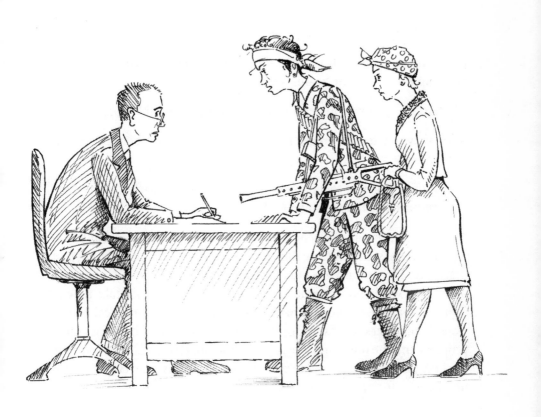

7. Common dilemmas faced by parent campaigners

In our discussions with parents, there are two interlinked themes that come up time and time again. These are:

1. Do we go for short-term warfare or long-term diplomacy?

And, if two sets of parents in one area respond differently to that question:

2. Is there a danger that parents using different approaches in the same authority will undermine each other?

This section sets out different viewpoints on these dilemmas, but PACE does not necessarily endorse the views expressed – nor do we think that there are simple answers. Our 'customised campaigning' approach means that we do not rule out any one approach, and it may take time to figure out which of two approaches is most appropriate to local conditions. In many cases the work in the case studies featured below is still in progress and the outcomes are as yet unknown. PACE plans to continue tracking parents' efforts and to update our learning as it develops – check our website for progress reports.

Do we go for short-term warfare or long-term diplomacy?

Two parent groups have taken very different approaches to this dilemma. For the first group, one parent describes their efforts in military language:

> Most people are attacking the wrong target and wasting their time. On the whole anyone who works on the council should be seen as the enemy by parents… Need is never the main criterion for deciding what will be paid for. They will never admit this because it would be breaking the law. You are in a war about money.

This parent applied two tactics. He learned that the council was conduct-ing two reviews of services, and he set up parent groups to respond to these reviews. At the same time he applied political pressure by encour-aging the parents to get to know councillors by taking part in local political party ward meetings. He believed that this would make council-lors feel vulnerable to de-selection.

Ultimately this parent went to SENDIST for his own child and achieved the funding for his home programme in an 'eleventh-hour' set-tlement with the LEA. To use his terminology, he clearly 'won' his own child's battle, but it is less clear whether he won the 'war' – that is, whether his individual success helped or hindered other families coming after him. Whether one agrees or not with his analysis of the problems, and his attempt to apply political pressure, his research and use of council procedures is an approach that other parents might find productive.

In contrast, another group of parents has chosen to work by support-ing their authority. Eight years ago they decided to get involved with local service-providers in order to help smooth the way through the process for other parents. One parent describes the work that this group has done for many years, building strong relationships with caseworkers and managers in order to help parents through the system, and through these links influencing how services are provided.

> We're all over them like a rash – networking and working with
> professionals to help parents get round the logjams, we're often more
> informed than the professionals are about what is going on; and we're
> good at helping parents to talk to the authority.

This parent feels that her group has achieved a great deal, and that awareness and provision for autism is far better than it was when her child was first diagnosed, but at times she is concerned that her group is manipulated by local service-providers.

> At times you feel you are being used and not getting deep change…
> You feel that you're selling yourself to the devil. For instance they have
> tried to use us to endorse a particular provision, to get other parents to
> have confidence in the service.

Nevertheless she feels that their approach has been effective:

> Just being there, just being a presence matters, it does something.
> When my child was diagnosed someone advised me, 'Be the dripping
> tap.' It might be tedious, it might be time-consuming, but it gives you a
> better chance of being listened to.

These cases illustrate dilemmas over style of approach – whether to confront or to try to work together with public authorities; and analysis of the problems – to what extent the roots of the problems faced by parents are at national or local level, and where best they can be tackled.

Several groups of parents have argued that the frequent conflict between parents and agencies at local level is largely the effect of deficiencies at national level, e.g. about lack of resources. They feel that parents need to address these issues through public campaigning at national level, and that it is unhelpful to hold local public authorities responsible for the limited resources and systemic problems that hamper them in carrying out their work.

These parents believe that the energy and resources of local authority officers is better spent developing strategic, long-term solutions to the problems on the ground, than defensively fighting parents and covering up for poor practice. While these solutions cannot solve problems caused by lack of funding, they can sometimes show local public agencies how to use available money more efficiently; they may attract extra funding by proposing creative solutions; and, by improving families' satisfaction with services, they cut the significant costs of fighting legal battles. They may even elicit a joint approach to national government from parents and professionals together.

Most parents grapple with this dilemma. Many seek to develop initiatives that avoid the twin dangers of alienating and colluding with public agencies. Over time some parents have changed their analysis of the problems, and the style of their approach.

One group of parents describes how, over time, they have changed their analysis of the problems facing their children, and how they have changed their approach to working for better provision for their children as a result. Initially they involved national media in highlighting their local problems.

In July 2002 Newsnight ran a well-researched and well-argued exposé of LEA failure to meet the needs of children with autism. It came about as a result of one of the parents in the group, who contacted the BBC about the problems faced by children with autism in her area. It opened with footage of parents describing the lack of provision for their children.

But these same parents now feel that the roots of the problems are at national level, and that they result both from a lack of resources, and poor planning for use of SEN resources in Wales. The parents have taken a dual strategy. They are contributing to efforts at national level to develop a strategy for autism in Wales, and they are working constructively and closely with their local authority. Targeting the LEA in a very public way had in fact created its own barriers and misconceptions.

> We had to build some fences after Newsnight, and we've realised that they are battling just as hard as we are to improve things, but they are very constrained in what they can say. I know a lot more now. They are in a very stressful position. We've realised that they're not ogres. The head of SEN has acknowledged what a huge problem there is for children with autism. We've drafted policy with the local authority and set up a local planning group with parents and representatives from education, health, social services and leisure, which have never really done any joint planning before. The group is in its infancy but it's really a step in the right direction.

As a result of working with the parents the authority has decided to expand the local autism school, and has worked out a way to do this without closing the local SLD (severe learning disability) school. They have also managed to access funds to develop autism units in mainstream schools, although at the moment, no schools have yet agreed to go ahead with this proposal.

Is there a danger that different parent approaches will undermine each other?

In one local authority individual parents and parent groups used different methods to raise awareness of various issues facing families affected by autism. Two parents' groups worked 'inside' the local authority and several individual parents campaigned 'outside' public agency structures. Of the latter, one family went to the press, contacted national politicians and even went on hunger strike, while another parent wrote leaflets asking the public to write to government ministers about her son's exclusion from school. The local press featured the issues prominently, but did not always seek the agreement of the parents concerned.

One of the 'insider' parents' groups was concerned about a general lack of provision for children with autism, and a lack of understanding of the particular challenges of including children with autism in mainstream school classrooms. This group took a decision to advise parents to contact local councillors about their children's problems. Another group sought local authority support for intensive early intervention programmes for pre-school children.

Following this activity, the council took an important decision to set up a scrutiny of provision for children with autism. This was a landmark for the authority: it meant that there would be a process of learning about autism to make informed decisions about future services. The scrutiny committee researched best autism practice and held 29 meetings, 17 of which were visits to different kinds of provision in different parts of the country. A series of recommendations was drawn up by the officers and councillors, in consultation with parent groups, all of which the council has agreed to implement. The existing autism liaison group in the authority was charged with monitoring implementation of the scrutiny group's recommendations, and officers and parents worked closely to ensure that the group would be constituted in such a way that everyone would trust its effectiveness.

There were different kinds of conflicts between the different parents and parent groups. The two parent groups had different objectives. Unlike a single-issue campaign which can unite a community, like trying to stop a new road being built, children with autism need different kinds of provision at different stages and according to where they are on the autism spectrum. It is a particular challenge for parents of children with autism to work together and overcome conflicts of interests over what they believe should be funding priorities.

The two groups acknowledge that this was a difficult process. Independently both established good working relationships with different senior managers within the authority, and during the scrutiny they put the merits of their different positions to councillors at separate meetings. But both groups recognised the importance of overcoming their different interests, and found a way to operate together at a key point in the process of change.

There were also conflicts between the two groups and the individual parents who were campaigning 'outside' the authority. Both groups were determined that the relationships with senior figures within the authority should be professional, effective and friendly. Neither group felt able to include the very stressed parents who were featured in the press in their discussions with the local authority, which at the time left some of the parents concerned feeling very let down. However, one of these parents now acknowledges the real gains made by the 'insider' parents and the scrutiny decisions, which include concrete plans to develop two units for children with autism in mainstream schools.

What brought about the scrutiny? Personal contacts that parents made with councillors, and hence the fact that they learned at first hand of the problems, created an informed group within the council that was concerned about autism. The vice-chair of the scrutiny topic group, one of the parent governor representatives on the council, played a key role. She says that getting to know one of the autism parents, and a chance visit to her home, made her realise just how hard the situation was for this parent and her child. This contact made her determined to do something about autism. She does not feel that the press coverage played any role in influencing either her or council members.

One important lesson from this case study is that it may be effective for different groups of parents to take different approaches within the same authority. Parents who establish working relationships with local authority officers do not always recognise that parents who take a more adversarial approach may provide a strong incentive to officers to develop solutions. Similarly, parents who take a more adversarial approach do not always recognise that parent groups that have established working relationships with the local authority may be achieving a great deal – providing officers with a legitimate process for change – despite appearances that little is happening. Real progress has been made in the authority as a result of the autism scrutiny, although it will take time, political will and a persistent parent presence for the recommended changes to be fully implemented.

These parents learned about local authority procedures and structures over time, in the course of their campaigning. The next chapter outlines some key aspects of what they and other parents have learned about how local authorities work.

8. Local government – structures, people and processes

This section outlines some of the relevant facts about how local government operates in England and Wales. It may be useful to know some of this background in order to target your work most effectively and increase your confidence and credibility. However, do not feel it is necessary to become an expert on local government before getting started – you will pick up most of the important information as you go along, and lots of the people who work within these structures themselves admit to being baffled by their complexity.

Funding

Local authorities have four main sources of income:

- *Central government grants*, based on the cost of providing a standard level of services, make up 48 per cent.

- *Council tax* raises 25 per cent; the upper limits are set by central Government.

- *Business rates* or *non domestic rates* are set and pooled by central government and then distributed to authorities. This makes up about 25 per cent.

- The rest comes from *direct charges for services*.

Decisions about the majority of resources available to local authorities are made by central government on the basis of a fixed formula. How the budget is divided up locally is to some extent decided by the relevant executive councillor or deputy, with advice from officers and subsequent ratification by the cabinet. Councils have very little power over their spending limits. Any discretion lies in making cuts, not increases. Parents who wish to lobby for more public resources for autism services need to tackle this at national level, not at local level.

Councils do, however, have great power in setting priorities within their financial limits: they are not allocated a fixed sum of funds to spend on autism services. There is thus considerable scope for parents to raise the profile of autism and the extent to which it is a priority on the local political agenda, by demonstrating the severity of need associated with autism, and the evidence for increasing numbers of children needing services.

Authorities vary widely in their vision and mechanisms for funding services. For instance, even as far back as 2001, one local authority in Wales found the means to combine education, health and social services funding for a specialist early intervention home-based education programme for a child with autism. As far as PACE knows, this was the first example of 'tripartite funding' (i.e. the three services all contributing resources) for a pre-school child with autism in the UK and we are still not aware of any other occasion in which this has happened.

Local government structure

In Scotland, Wales, London or the English Metropolitan areas, most of the functions of local government are carried out by a unitary authority, usually known as a borough council. These are in significantly populated areas and have just one tier of government. In the rest of England there are two major tiers of local government – the large county council and the smaller district councils.

In April 2001 the Local Government Act 2000 came into force, dramatically changing the political structure of local government. The old committee system was abolished and replaced by separate decision-making and scrutiny bodies, with different elected members assigned to each. The structure is now more like central government, with cabinet ministers making decisions while other elected members check or 'scrutinise' their activities. Power has been shifted from large committees to a small number of executive councillors.

The Local Government Act created two new types of councillor:

- *Executive councillors* – councillors who are allocated a specific area of responsibility, and who are legally able to make certain decisions without approval of a committee or the council. They are chosen by the ruling political party, and collectively make up the cabinet.

- *Non-executive councillors* – councillors who are not party to decision-making. In the new system, they have a key role in scrutinising the work of the executive members of the council.

This is a fundamental change in British local government, because it creates a political executive, or a cabinet, separate from the council as a whole. However, all councillors are duty bound to act as advocates for the electorate in their ward. Many councillors run advice surgeries, make home visits or will talk on the phone. They should be able to give advice or tell you whom to contact to deal with your particular problem. Furthermore, all councillors have a specified area of interest. They may relate to a locality or a particular issue.

Under the previous system community and voluntary sector groups were represented by the committee system. To continue to be represented effectively, these groups need to take an active role in policy formation groups and on scrutiny panels, which then feed into decision-making.

Who's who in local government?

Local authorities are run by councillors, who are elected by local people to make decisions and set policies, and a permanent staff of officers who are paid to advise councillors and implement policies. Councillors receive an allowance and expenses, and usually have other paid work; officers are salaried and hold non-political positions.

In practice officers do most of the day-to-day work of running the local authority. However, it is important to remember that they are the agents of the council and are constrained by the council's decisions.

The leader of the council is the head of the political group with the most seats on the council. Political power is centred on the leader's office. Where there is no outright majority it is known as a 'hung council'. Coalitions of parties may be formed giving a clear majority and some political stability to the council. Where there is a hung council you need to pay attention to all the main parties, not just the controlling group. In theory a hung council increases the potential for influence from outsiders.

In most local authorities the leader is elected by the council, and the cabinet is made up of councillors, either appointed by the leader or elected by the council. In some authorities a mayor is elected by the whole electorate, and the mayor then selects a cabinet from among the councillors. The cabinet can be drawn from a single party or a coalition. In a small number of local authorities there may be a slightly different constitution.

The chief executive of a local authority is the head of all paid staff or officers. The chief executive's department has the job of co-ordinating the policy of the whole council. Small units like equality units and grant units, if they exist, are usually found in the chief executive's department. In many authorities the chief executive also holds the post of monitoring officer. This job is to ensure that the authority's decisions or actions do not break the law or constitute improper practice.

In authorities which have not yet begun to introduce the changes to services described in *Every Child Matters* (Department for Education and Skills 2003a, 2004a, 2004b) (see Chapter 9, p.93), the departments of education and social services have been run separately, and each is headed by a chief officer, usually known as a director. Health provision come under separate NHS structures – see Chapter 9.

Under the changes each council will have to appoint a new director of children's services, accountable for all the children's services functions of the local authority i.e. for both education and children's social services. In Wales this post will be described as the lead director for children's and youth services. The director of children's services will also be responsible for the local authority's children's trust, the body that brings together resources and budgets for education, children's social services, some children's health services and the Connexions service, as well as partners in the voluntary and community sectors.

Councils will have to appoint a lead member who will hold political responsibility for local child welfare. This will mean that local groups will have a single point of contact with whom to raise their concerns. Prior to the appointment of a single lead member for children, different councillors may take different areas of responsibility for children's services.

In some local authorities this change is beginning to take place. In one local authority, for instance, education and children's social services have been brought together into a single Children, Schools and Families department. Different local authorities have always organised responsibilities within their departments in different ways, depending on their local circumstances. Particular groups may be set up to pursue a particular goal. For instance, in another LEA a multi-agency strategy group was set up to bring together heads of different services to develop a practical inclusion policy.

Using local authority structures
The formalities of decision-making

Local authorities are now required to publish a forward plan. It should set out key decisions to be taken in the next four months. It should be updated monthly and give details of who is dealing with the issue and any arrangements for consultation.

The executive is responsible for the effective implementation of council policy and delivering services in line with the council's approved budget and policy framework. Decisions can be taken by the whole cabinet, in sub-groups or in combinations of these. Cabinets may have between six to a dozen members and portfolios can be a mixture of service-based (e.g. education) and cross-cutting remits (e.g. children and families).

Cabinet meetings are held in cycles which vary but are usually every six weeks, culminating in a meeting of the full council at which cabinet decisions are finally approved or not. All these meetings are open to the public.

All 'key' decisions must be made public and agendas, officers' reports and background papers, which are not in the forward plan, must be available at least three days in advance. This does not apply to items classified as exempt information.

There is no agreement on what is a 'key' decision, or on what distinguishes major decisions and day-to-day management decisions. Executives can meet and take decisions in private without the requirement to publish relevant papers in advance. However, details of all executive decisions, whether made in private or in public, must be published afterwards with the relevant background papers.

All councillors have rights of access to documents in the possession of executive members. Under the Freedom of Information Act 2000 the public and media have access rights to all information held by the council, unless it is covered by the exemptions in the Act. If information is withheld you can appeal to the Information Commissioner, who can make the council publish the information.

Supporting structures

A number of advisory structures support executive decision-making. A cabinet member may have several advisory groups. For instance, the education portfolio holder may have 'lead members' with a deputy role, supporting different areas of policy, although the executive member retains overall responsibility. Education sub-committees are sometimes still in place to advise the executive. These structures allow the executive to share an enormous workload and are likely to survive, even if their power base has been redefined by the new legislation. There may also be advisory groups and external involvement from consultative groups, forums and taskforces.

Local government mechanisms that parents can use
Overview and scrutiny committees

Parents' groups can usefully contribute to a scrutiny process, and indeed make a case to councillors of the benefits of a time-limited scrutiny panel to look at autism or SEN generally.

All councils must have one or more overview and scrutiny committee. They are made up of councillors who are not members of the executive or cabinet and reflect the political balance of the authority. Their meetings are open to the public and their recommendations are published.

Scrutiny is intended to ensure that councils are fulfilling all their legal obligations. Its role is:

- to review and develop the council's policies
- to make policy and budget proposals to the council
- to review proposed executive decisions
- to call in or review decisions before they are implemented
- to monitor performance
- to scrutinise other local organisations, including health services.

Councils can choose whether to have different scrutiny committees for particular services, such as education or the environment, or whether to have only one scrutiny body, which ensures that *all* the council's services are scrutinised. There must also be a scrutiny body that looks at local health service issues, and possibly other public services that are not run by the council itself.

The remit and structure of scrutiny activities is very broad and changes over time. They may mirror executive portfolios (e.g. an education scrutiny panel) or they may be more thematic (e.g. a social inclusion scrutiny panel). The statutory guidance is that they should take a 'cross-cutting' or thematic rather than a narrow service-based view.

The cabinet decides the remit and scope of a council's scrutiny panels. They are intended to enable councillors to learn the views of their electorate. Some will call external witnesses, or make visits to provision within and outside the authority.

Some councils show a real commitment to ensuring that scrutiny leads to changes in policy. Very positive developments in one county have come from the setting up of a scrutiny specifically on autism provision (see Chapter 7).

> [The scrutiny has] provided us with an invaluable set of priorities and actions for development over the next five years… The benefits are enormous in clarifying issues; celebrating good practice and developing the right framework for future development. It also gave us a chance to look at what other LEAs were doing in this area. (Local authority senior officer)

SCRUTINY TEMPLATE

This is a very helpful guide for parents, produced by IPSEA, a leading SEN advice and advocacy organisation (see the Resources section for contact details). You can access it on www.ipsea.org.uk/scrutinyreview.htm.

As a note of caution, however, one parent who is very experienced in the local government process highlights that having a scrutiny process is not the end of the story:

> The hard part is to follow through relentlessly. Officers feel that after the [scrutiny] committee has risen, they're done. 'Phew, through that.' That's when the hard work starts, otherwise it will be, 'Autism? We did that last year.'

Questions

Many councils have question sessions with executive councillors. Parents who have built relationships with backbench councillors can place specific questions with these councillors to ask the relevant executive councillor. The executive councillor will expect the officers to be able to provide the answers to such questions, and this process may reveal gaps in the council's knowledge around autism that you can use in your campaigning.

Standards committees

Every council in England and Wales must set up a standards committee, which has at least one independent or lay member, with the function of promoting and maintaining high standards of conduct in the authority. You may wish to approach this committee if you are unhappy with the professional conduct of councillors or officers – but again, you need to think about the likely impact of this on your existing relationships – it is probably only a 'last ditch' mechanism.

Using the auditing process

Accounts are audited every year and the auditor sets a date when local people can ask questions.

Find out from the council finance department when this date is. For 15 days before that date there is a public right to inspect the accounts and all documents relating to them. You might be able to compare actual spending to the budget. In such a short period of time and given the difficulty of knowing what to look for, it's unlikely that you'll make a conclusive case but that doesn't necessarily matter. This is a good time to raise questions to the auditor, who might investigate further.

A large part of the auditor's job is to assess 'value for money'. This tends to be based on accounting figures rather than experience of the services, so they rely heavily on the public to bring issues of concern to their attention, particularly on efficiency and performance.

Alongside an understanding of local authority structures, people and processes outlined in this chapter, it is important to plan your campaigning in the light of how children's services are changing. This is the subject of the next chapter.

9. Changes to children's services [1]

Policy and structures

There are major changes taking place in the way that children's services are organised in England and Wales. It is important to understand a little about these changes, because they create new opportunities for parents to influence the development of autism services.

> *In your conversations and letters demonstrate an awareness of central government policy, new research and what other LEAs are doing. If you show that you understand the current policy issues you will be less likely to be fobbed off.*

How education, social services and health fit together

Prior to the changes at national level, responsibility for education was held by a separate government department to health and social services. At local level, responsibility for each department was exercised separately, and only education and social services were run by locally elected councils.

Since the changes, in England, government responsibility for both education and children's social services is now exercised through the Department for Education and Skills. Children's health services continue to be the responsibility of the Department of Health (DoH). In Wales, responsibility for all children's services is devolved to the Welsh Assembly, though the Assembly does not have the power to make primary legislation or to raise taxes.

---

1   For further information about all the documents and policies referred to in this chapter, please see the Resources section at the end of the Handbook.

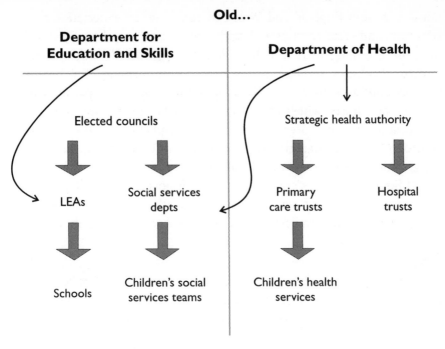

Figure 9.1 Traditional structure for children's services

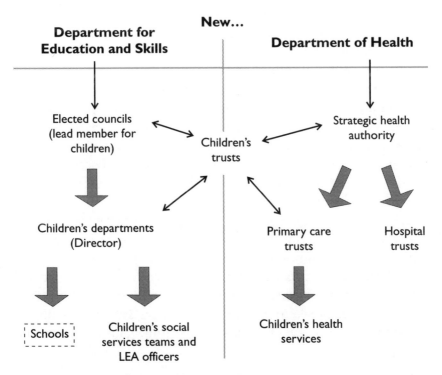

Figure 9.2 Emerging structure for children's services

Locally, in both England and Wales, there is now an expectation that education and social services will work more closely together and structures are changing to reflect this, often through the development of unified children's services departments. Responsibility for health services continues to be exercised by separate agencies, particularly primary care trusts, which are under the management of the strategic health authority, and over which local government has only limited control. Often the strategic health authority does not share the same geographical boundaries as the local council.

Although structures are still separate, all government policy statements are urging closer working between health, education and social services, and mechanisms have been developed to bring this about.

Education

Local education authorities are part of the structure of your local council and are accountable to elected members. LEAs have responsibility for providing education services for school-age children and pre-school early intervention.

Increasingly, however, schools themselves are receiving funding directly to provide for children with SEN ('delegated funding'), and school governing bodies have important responsibilities to plan and deliver SEN support. The policy direction is for schools to have much greater autonomy than has been the case to date, and also that they will be used as bases for the provision of other services.

Local education authorities are expected to develop a more strategic role as funding is increasingly delegated to schools, though the implementation of this varies from authority to authority. In some areas LEAs are becoming a specialist support service for schools, providing a forward-looking strategic base rather than operational services. LEAs do however continue to have legal responsibility for organising and delivering provision for all children with a statement of SEN.

Schools have a duty to publish an SEN policy which must contain a wide range of information, from how the school is meeting its accessibility planning duty to how resources are allocated to pupils without statements. LEAs have a parallel duty to publish an accessibility strategy which looks at how all the provision in the LEA will be made more accessible for disabled pupils. More information on accessibility planning is contained in the Resources section – see Department for Education and Skills 2000.

The government is moving to give schools ever-greater freedom to run their own affairs. Although this may bring benefits, PACE is concerned that it may mean that schools will be less motivated to meet the needs of children who don't fulfil the 'standards agenda' (exam results), and that they will have an incentive to exclude or ignore children who are seen to be a drain on resources. Added to that, delegating funding straight to schools potentially reduces the role of the LEA and 'hides' where the SEN funds are spent. For children with statements of SEN, it can also lead to the bizarre situation where the school has the money to support their child, but the LEA retains the legal responsibility when things go wrong.

Parents of children with SEN might play a significant role as school governors in mainstream schools to which SEN funds have largely been delegated, providing that they do not confine their interests to children with SEN alone. PACE is keen to learn of parents who are developing expertise in this area – please contact us if you are taking this role.

Social services

As with education, social services departments are part of the structure of an elected council. Most local authorities still have a single social services department providing social care support for both children and adults. However, as mentioned above, there is a key change underway to unify education and social care for children within a single department. Although this is positive in organising services for children, it may make it harder to plan and organise the period of transition to adult social care services. Within children's social services, most local authorities have distinct teams covering different areas – looked after children, children with disabilities, child and adolescent mental health services (CAMHS),[2] etc. Some families find that the needs of children with autism are ignored because they do not fit neatly into these structures.

A growing role for social services departments is the administration of direct payments, cash payments made to families in place of services that would traditionally be provided by the local authority. There are

---

2   CAMHS are generally made up of health and social services staff, and subject
       to local variations as to which authority structure they fall within. Several will
       fall within the structure of the health service primary care trusts.

substantial differences in approach to direct payments between authorities, and parent campaigners should look into whether they are being made available to families affected by autism, as this is potentially an excellent unifying issue for campaigning.

There is growing scope for parents to influence how social care services are delivered to meet the needs of young people with autism. This is because of initiatives like the National Service Framework for Children (see below), and through the bringing together of responsibility for children's services in the newly created posts of director of children's services and lead cabinet member for children's services. The individuals taking these posts will hold ultimate responsibility for services for children with autism, and can therefore be held to account by parents.

Health

Primary care trusts are the cornerstone of the NHS. Overall, they are responsible for the health of the people in their area, tackling health inequalities and bringing health and social care more closely together. Each PCT holds about 75 per cent of the total NHS budget for its local area.

The role of a primary care trust is to:

- support and develop the services of GPs and their practice teams

- provide a range of community health services, such as health visiting and district nursing

- commission hospital treatment and specialist care for patients.

While acute care is provided by hospital and ambulance trusts, mental health services – including CAMHS – are provided by community trusts, now known generally as NHS and social care trusts, to reflect their closer working arrangements with colleagues from social services departments. Along with mental health, these trusts also provide social care assistance, such as help for people with disabilities, addiction services, and help for people with eating disorders.

The strategic health authority is responsible for identifying the health needs of local people and arranging for services to be provided by hospitals, doctors (via primary care trusts) and others.

Its role includes:

- making sure local NHS trusts are performing well
- improving the quality and consistency of health services in the local area
- making sure national health programmes are put into place locally.

Recent reforms have given an important scrutiny function over local health services to elected local councillors. This may make it easier for parents to influence the workings of local health authorities, although at the time of writing these arrangements are still evolving.

Bringing the services together: recent government policy

In the last few years the direction of central government policy has been to try to integrate the work of all three services: health, education and social care. Policy-making is now focused on co-ordinating services and on putting people's needs first, rather than letting priorities be determined by organisational structures. In particular, there has been a drive to integrate services around the needs of children and their families. The emphasis is on earlier detection of problems and ensuring that responsibility does not slip between different agencies. This has been driven largely by child protection concerns, but as there is a recognition that child protection cannot be separated from policies to improve children's lives as a whole, the changes are far-reaching and have the potential to have significant impact for children with disabilities.

The government's Green Paper *Every Child Matters* (Department for Education and Skills 2003), and the subsequent *Next Steps* (Department for Education and Skills 2004b), have brought together the ideas being developed in many existing and proposed initiatives for integrating services. They tackle the ways that services are located, managed, funded and held accountable.

Key features of Every Child Matters
JOINT WORKING BY PROFESSIONALS

On the ground the aim is for professionals from education, social services and health increasingly to work together, for instance in extended schools and children's centres. This is already happening in some areas, for instance through Sure Start and child development centres.

BETTER INFORMATION SHARING

Integration is also the intention behind moves to improve information sharing between agencies and professionals, to provide a common assessment framework that professionals from different disciplines will use together, and for children and families who receive a number of different services to have a lead professional to ensure that services are coherent.

BETTER ALLOCATION OF RESOURCES

One problem with separate departments has been that each held control of its own budget. Sometimes this meant that the needs of an individual child or family would be lost in inter-departmental arguments over who was going to pay for what. And each agency would seek to meet only its own immediate obligations; it was not in the interests of the individual departments to address the long-term outcomes for children and families.

To address this, children's trusts are to be introduced to pool budgets and resources, and integrate the commissioning of services. The idea is that this will enable agencies to work together at strategic level to develop services that achieve better long-term outcomes for children and families as a whole. Children's trusts will be accountable to local government.

The government proposes that children's trusts should be set up in most areas by 2006, and in all areas by 2008. Thirty-five children's trusts have been set up in 2004 to pilot the proposals. There is a lot of flexibility in the form these will take organisationally, and what they will prioritise, depending on local circumstances. Ofsted will take the lead responsibility for inspecting all children's services to assess how successfully they are being integrated.

One of the problematic areas in the new reforms is that while they address how to bring health, education and social care together, they do not clarify how schools, with much greater autonomy and responsibilities than before, will fit into the new structures. Concerns about the accountability of schools have been raised above. It may make sense for parent campaigners to find ways to work at school-based level, perhaps by developing links with school governors, and school governor representatives on local councils.

Other key policy documents
THE CHILDREN'S NATIONAL SERVICE FRAMEWORK

In parallel to *Every Child Matters*, discussed above, the government has published the Children's National Service Framework (NSF), a set of standards based on a vision of seamless, family-centred services (Department of Health and Department for Education and Skills 2004a, 2004b). Autism is at the heart of this crucial initiative – there is an exemplar 'care pathway' to guide service delivery for children with autism in an important appendix to the Disabled Children's Module. This section was informed by the *National Autism Plan for Children* (NAP-C) (NIASA 2003), a set of standards for diagnosis, assessment and early intervention produced by an independent expert working party. Some local public agencies are looking at how to implement the NAP-C standards, which in some ways are more ambitious than the government's vision in the NSF.

REMOVING BARRIERS TO ACHIEVEMENT

Removing Barriers to Achievement (Department for Education and Skills 2004c) is the government's Strategy for SEN, which sets out a ten-year vision for schools and local authorities. This puts forward ways to ensure that every child with SEN gets an appropriate education and child-care support, and that every parent is satisfied with the provision made for his or her child. The strategy builds on the *Report of the Special Schools Working Group* (Department for Education and Skills 2003b) to give a clear message that special schools are an important part of what the then minister, Baroness Ashton, referred to as an 'inclusive education system' (pp34–38).

There are two key areas that parents may wish to focus on, as they have specific relevance to children with autism:

1. *Early intervention*: significant funds have been invested in services for very young disabled children.

2. *Training/workforce reform*: a recognition that there needs to be more specialist staff, and that individuals who work with children need training to support children with SEN and disabilities.

Four common misinterpretations of government policy

They over-complicate stuff, blame the legislation; but actually it often turns out that they've misinterpreted it themselves.

Parents report that local authorities frequently quote government policy inaccurately or selectively. Sometimes these assertions are an attempt to pass off unpopular local decisions as implementation of government policy. It is important that parents have an accurate understanding of the current position as stated by the government, so that they can rebut inaccurate statements of policy. The following are the most frequent questionable interpretations of government policy.

1. *'It is government policy to close special schools.'*
    Incorrect. The government's Strategy for SEN states that special schools have a crucial role to play in educating children with 'severe and complex needs' and in sharing their expertise with mainstream schools to promote meaningful inclusion. This should be supported by greater staff and pupil movement between special and mainstream schools. The Strategy states that 'local authorities have an important strategic role to play in planning a spectrum of provision needed to meet children's needs within their area' (p37).

2. *'The government's vision of inclusion means putting all children with SEN in a mainstream school.'*
    Incorrect. While the rights of all children with SEN to attend a mainstream school have been set out in legislation, this is not the same thing as forcing children into mainstream schools. The government recognises that:

    -   some children with autism can have a more 'inclusive' experience in specialist provision

    -   that there will need to be considerable effort in *all* settings to enable a child with autism to have an inclusive experience, through resourced support from well-trained staff, and this may embrace flexibility between more than one school and home.

3. *'It is already government policy to reduce the number of Statements.'*
    Correct – but only with parental support. You should never take at face value the simple assertion that a wholesale reduction in statements is government policy. The SEN Strategy is clear that attempts to reduce reliance on statements must involve a 'strong partnership' with parents. It states that reducing statements 'must result in a better deal for children and their parents, not reduced entitlements' (p.18). It points out that where this has not happened,

'reductions in statements have given rise to great anxiety and confusion' amongst parents' (pp.18–19).

It is absolutely crucial to understand that the government has not changed the SEN legal framework. Recent reports by the Audit Commission and the Cabinet Office have recommended that the DfES consider changing the law on SEN, but so far this recommendation has been rejected. Although the SEN Strategy encourages schools to meet children's needs without statements where possible, parents have the right to request an assessment, and can appeal to SENDIST on specific issues relating to the statutory assessment and statementing process. Ministers are clear that an LEA that claims no longer to be issuing statements is acting unlawfully.

LEAs are legally obliged to take all the factors of an individual case into account so it is unlawful for them to adopt blanket policies.

4. *'It is government policy to delegate all SEN funds to schools.'*
   Incorrect. The SEN Strategy endorses the policy of local education authorities delegating SEN funds directly to schools, as this is seen to support early intervention, but does not state that this should apply to *all* SEN funds. PACE has concerns about delegation of funding, and the SEN Strategy itself emphasises that delegation must take place in the context of better monitoring and accountability of schools by LEAs. Significantly, the DfES has now withdrawn fixed delegation targets for LEAs, recognising concerns about their potential impact on SEN support services.

These misinterpretations highlight the sensitivities in the relationship between parents, local agencies and national government policy. Maximum campaigning effectiveness will be achieved by parents who have an understanding of both local and national agendas. National voluntary organisations such as TreeHouse, the National Autistic Society, Contact a Family and the Council for Disabled Children all regularly update their websites and information sheets with bulletins on changes in government policy. The key government website for policy changes affecting children with autism is www.dfes.gov.uk/sen. For further sources of information, please see the Resources section.

The new national policy initiatives and the misinterpretations of government policy described above are both responses to the tensions currently inherent in autism services, examined in the next chapter.

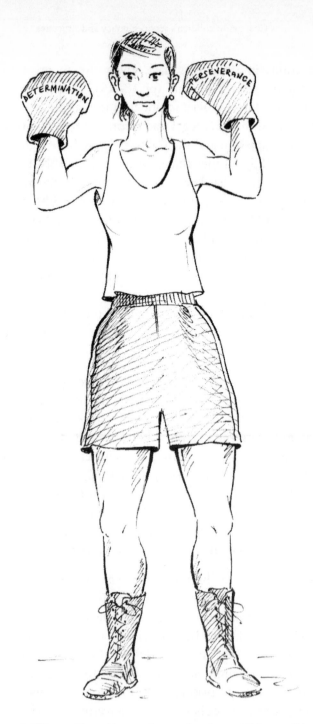

'The parents of children with autism are the two-fisted street fighters of the disability movement.'

— Dr Stephen Ladyman MP, February 2002
Autism Awareness Year Conference, King's Fund, London

10. The current state of autism services

Parents should be inspired by and proud of their part in the progress that has been made for children with autism since the 1960s. But we will also inevitably be outraged and indignant on those occasions when agencies continue to fail in their responsibilities towards some of the most vulnerable members of our society.

Making further improvements happen as quickly as possible requires an understanding of the obstacles as well as the opportunities – and being familiar with the context in which we are all working.

An Audit Commission report on disabled children's services stated:

> The time for a major turnaround in disabled children's services is long overdue. The urgency of the situation is growing. Not only are some services provided at unacceptably low standards, but the prevalence of certain needs is increasing. Without change the situation can only get worse. (Audit Commission 2003, p.11)

Autism has only been recognised very recently, and is still poorly understood. In 1960, barely anyone knew what autism was; in 1990, few people had heard of Asperger syndrome; and until very recently, autism was not on the radar of politicians and policy-makers. In 2001, a health minister told a fellow MP who had put a House of Commons question about the number of people affected by autism that:

> Not only do we not know how many people are affected by the condition, but before you put the question, we did not know that we did not know.

Against this back-cloth of widespread ignorance about autism, there has been a dramatic increase in the numbers of children being diagnosed: since the mid-1990s accepted prevalence rates of autism spectrum disorders have increased tenfold. In 2001 the Medical Research Council estimated that one child in 166 children under eight had autism. Teachers surveyed in a NAS report in 2002, *Autism in Schools: Crisis or Challenge?* (Barnard *et al.* 2002), reported that 1 in 86 children they taught had an autistic spectrum disorder.

It is hardly surprising, therefore, that children with autism so often receive poor services: only very recently have public bodies known the scale of the challenge, let alone begun to invest in provision and training to meet the need. Different authorities have responded to the problems in very different ways, resulting in a 'postcode lottery' for children and families. Variations stem from genuine differences of professional and parental opinion about the most appropriate settings and approaches for teaching children with autism, shifting political priorities and, in some authorities, a lack of vision and ignorance of autism that leads to simplified 'solutions' that do not take into account the specific needs of individual children.

The result of all this is:

- a shortfall in skills and specialist provision
- pressure on parents and families
- conflict between parents and local public agencies.

The shortfall in skills and specialist provision

Children of every age with autism need access to people who will teach them in ways that address their unique differences – in areas such as sensory and information processing, communication and social interaction. But there is a huge shortfall in autism-specific provision, skills and awareness. For an estimated 90,000 children with autism there are just 7,500 specialist school places (Jones 2002). Even if three-quarters of children with autism were able to access mainstream schools, an arbitrary and very ambitious figure, two out of three of the remaining children would not have access to the specialist provision they need.

According to one report, among the 70 per cent of the teachers sampled who had worked with a child with autism, only 5 per cent had received any autism-specific training. According to the NAS (Barnard *et al.* 2002) survey, a fifth of schools with pupils with autism have no teachers with autism-specific training at all, and where there is some training this is usually cursory and only accessed by a fifth of the staff.

There is also a pressing need for greater autism awareness and training among early years staff and social workers, to enable them to identify children and make accurate assessments, and to provide autism-appropriate social and family care and support services. Within social services departments, lack of knowledge of the autism spectrum can lead to inappropriate questioning of parents' parenting skills, rather than recognising that children's behaviours are linked to their distinct neurological condition.

Pressure on parents and families

The result is that services for children with autism and their families are under massive pressure. Already very stretched by a challenging disability, families carry the brunt of a major systemic problem, and the cost of the stress that ensues is desperately high, leading some families to relationship breakdown, serious mental health problems or just straightforward despair. In a highly publicised case in 2001, one single mother of a child with autism killed herself and her son. In the absence of the support she needed, she had no confidence in a viable future: one in which she and her son would be able to stay together.

For parents who have the resources – inner strength, time and often money – the quest for the education and support they believe their children need will often take them to SENDIST. The annual increase in autism-related cases going to SENDIST highlights the danger that, far from improving, the problems posed by autism in some areas may actually be getting worse. PACE knows of many families that have decided that the only solution is to move to a different local authority, or to educate at home.

Conflict between parents and local public agencies

Parents are often infuriated by what they see as public authorities failing not only their child but other children too. They see authorities who have reacted defensively, resorting to evasion and delaying tactics in an effort to save funds. In such LEAs there are very poor relationships between the authority and parents.

One prominent policy expert in local government stated publicly at a conference in 2003 that she had never come across a policy area where there was so much mistrust as SEN. At the 2004 National Union of Teachers SEN conference, the responsible minister, Baroness Ashton, described parents of children with SEN as 'lost in a battleground for their child'.

Poor communication between many authorities and parents is made worse by a number of other structural problems. Key among these is a lack of co-ordinated services. Many parents despair at the institutional barriers they meet, and find that negotiating their way between them is a full-time job.

In recent years, the government (and in particular ministers and civil servants at the Department for Education and Skills) have been candid about some of the problems listed above, and the obstacles to providing appropriate services for all children with disabilities.

> SEN is one of the most difficult and challenging of local authorities' responsibilities…too often parents face a 'postcode lottery' in the support available from their school, local education authority and social services…a culture of mistrust has grown up in some areas, such that parents feel they need to 'fight' for the support to which their child is entitled. (Department for Education and Skills 2004c, p.71).

The policy documents outlined in the previous chapter set out the government's vision for solving these challenges. Parents need to be aware that the implementation of this vision at local level is not an automatic process, presenting challenges and tensions as well as opportunities for real progress.

Central government is increasingly reluctant to set specific milestones and targets for local agencies. So although the policy documents set clear standards for services, they still leave a large degree of autonomy to local agencies to interpret how the standards are implemented on the ground.

Some ministers have openly stated that there is simply not enough money in disabled children's services. PACE is very concerned at the difficulties that local agencies will have in delivering the government's vision for children with autism without significant new resources, and is working at national level to raise these concerns.

At local level the consequences of lack of funding for these initiatives are serious. As highlighted above, parents frequently report that local agencies misapply government policy. Parents often suspect that local authorities are taking a simplified view of government policy to disguise efforts to protect budgets and reduce expenditure.

When government sets policy and passes legislation, it is intended for roll-out at local level. Yet increasingly, the implementation of national policy is left very much to local discretion. Nationally set constraints, particularly in relation to resources, have huge impact on parents' experiences at local level.

But the difficulties themselves provide opportunities. For each obstacle there is a positive argument for change. The need for greater autism skills among professionals is an issue that unites everyone in the autism movement, and as such provides a compelling focus for campaigning. Because the facts presented above, and in Chapter 5 (see pp.54–56), are both so damning and so persuasive, and because they are supported by a whole series of reports and initiatives, there is a unique opportunity to build a head of steam for change through combined local and national campaigning. Similarly, with regard to the pressure on parents and families, if each family affected by autism and under pressure from the obstacles described above were to undertake just one of the activities set out in Chapter 4, this would generate thousands of communications to key decision-makers and this in turn would move autism up the political agenda. Parents are the best source of help to each other here, offering assistance and inspiration.

The communication of what has been learned in one local area can have significant influence in others: what you are doing locally may have wider impact. It is always worth sharing the successes, as well as the problems, that you have faced, as the many parents we have talked to have done in this handbook. PACE would like to hear of your experiences and your response to this handbook so that we can continue to inform parents of what we are all learning.

And potentially a very powerful role parents can play is in helping tired professionals become partners in awareness-raising. Imagine what could be done if each parent persuaded just one person from a public agency each year to alert someone higher up the system, or someone in national government, to the issues he or she was dealing with. Combined parent/professional lobbying stops the rot of 'divide and rule', and will also surprise anyone who is used to a more familiar battleground scenario.

All these are reasons why parents are so important. Parents are the experts on what their children need and the state of current services in their area. They can also be the most dynamic and effective agents for change. Thanks largely to parental effort, children with autism are no longer confined in institutions and labelled uneducable. But there is still a very long way to go. Customised campaigning by parents is vital so that all children with autism will finally get the services they need.

Resources

References and key documents

Please refer to the section 'Advisory organisations and contact details' for contact details for many of the organisations publishing the documents listed below.

All-Party Parliamentary Group on Autism (2001) *The Rising Challenge*. NAS 488. London: NAS. Available at www.nas.org.uk/pubs.

Audit Commission (2002) *Special Educational Needs: A Mainstream Issue*. London: Audit Commission.

Audit Commission (2003) *Services for Disabled Children*. London: Audit Commission
These two Audit Commission documents are very useful surveys of current provision. Both available at www.audit-commission.gov.uk.

Barnard, J., Prior, J. and Potter, D. (2000) *Inclusion and Autism: Is it Working?* London: NAS.

Barnard, J., Broach, S., Potter, D. and Prior, A. (2002) *Autism in Schools: Crisis or Challenge?* NAS450. London: NAS.

Contact a Family/Council for Disabled Children (2004) *Parent Participation: Improving Services for Disabled Children: Parents' Guide*. London: Contact a Family.
An essential resource for any parent wanting to work with their local authority. Available free at www.cafamily.org.uk/parentparticipationguide.pdf.

Department for Education and Skills (2002) *Accessible Schools: Summary Guidance*. DfES/0462/2002. Nottingham: DfES Publications.
Schools and LEAs have new legal duties to plan, in order to increase access for all disabled pupils – duties and guidance at at www.teachernet.gov.uk/wholeschool/sen/schools/accessibility/dda.

Department for Education and Skills (2003a) *Every Child Matters*. Nottingham: DfES Publications. Available at www.everychildmatters.gov.uk/publications

Department for Education and Skills (2003b) *Report of the Special Schools Working Group*. DfES/0258/2003. Nottingham: DfES Publications. Available at http://www.teachernet.gov.uk/wholeschool/sen/schools/specialschoolswg/

Department for Education and Skills (2004a) *Every Child Matters: Change for Children*. Nottingham: DfES Publications. Available at www.everychildmatters.gov.uk/publications

Department for Education and Skills (2004b) *Every Child Matters: Next Steps*. Nottingham: DfES Publications. Available at www.everychildmatters.gov.uk/publications
The current reforms to all children's services are set out in the policy paper *Every Child Matters* (DfES 2003a) and its successors (DfES 2004a, 2004b). The scope of the reforms is vast and parents will not need to know all the details, but reading the executive summaries can give you a useful overview of the key priorities for local agencies.

Department for Education and Skills (2004c) *Removing Barriers to Achievement: The Government's Strategy for SEN.* DfES/0117/2004. Nottingham: DfES Publications. Available at http://www.teachernet.gov.uk/wholeschool/sen/senstrategy/
The government's 10-year plan for improving SEN provision – crucial to any parent working with their LEA.

Department for Education and Skills/Department of Health (2002) *Autistic Spectrum Disorders Good Practice Guidance.* DfES/597/2002. Nottingham: DfES Publications. Available at http://www.teachernet.gov.uk/wholeschool/sen/ teacherlearningassistant/asd/
Practical and specific guidance to schools and LEAs on provision for children with autism. It includes examples of good practice that can be used to measure the quality of provision in your area, and to show that other areas may be doing more.

Department of Health and Department for Education and Skills (2004a) *National Service Framework for Children, Young People and Maternity Services: Core standards.* DH3779. London: DH Publications.

Department of Health and Department for Education and Skills (2004b) *National Service Framework for Children, Young People and Maternity Services: Disabled Children and Young People and those with Complex Health Needs.* DH3779. London: DH Publications. Available at www.dh.gov.uk. Access via the A to Z site index.
The NSF is the key initiative for reforming children's health services. The most relevant sections are the executive summary, the disabled children's module and the ASD exemplar, which gives an example of good practice service delivery to a child with autism.

House of Commons Information Office (2003) *You and Your MP.* Factsheet M1, Member's series. Available at www.parliament.uk/documents/upload/m01.pdf.

Jones, G. (2002) *Educational Provision for Children with Autism and Asperger Syndrome: Meeting Their Needs.* London: David Fulton Publishers.

Medical Research Council (2001) *Review of Autism Research: Causes and Epidemiology.* London: MRC. Available at www.mrc.ac.uk/pdf-autism-report.pdf
For parents interested in the current state of autism research. This also contains the 'official' prevalence rate of autism of 60 in 10,000 children under 8.

NIASA (National Initiative for Autism Screening and Assessment) (2003) *National Autism Plan for Children.* NAS 477. London: NAS. Available at www.nas.org.uk/pubs.
Very helpful expert guidelines for good practice in assessment and early intervention. Recommendations include minimum hours of intervention for pre-school children.

Legislation

Key pieces of legislation affecting children with autism include:

- Special Educational Needs and Disability Act 2001
- Carers and Disabled Children Act 2000
- Disability Discrimination Act 1995 (as amended)
- NHS and Community Care Act 1990
- Children Act 1989

All legislation can be found on the parliament website at www.opsi.gov.uk/acts.htm – use the search engine. However, reading Acts is very daunting, and if you want to find out about your legal rights you may wish to start by looking at the websites of the advisory organisations listed below.

Political resources

Along with the BBC Politics website (www.bbc.co.uk/politics), **Epolitix** (www.epolitix.com) is an excellent source of information on political developments.

A free, fast and easy way to **contact your MP** is to use the excellent www.FaxYourMP. com. A partner website to FaxYourMP is www.theyworkforyou.com, which has a wealth of information about your MP and how he or she votes in parliament.

The Information Commissioner is an independent official appointed by the Crown to oversee the Data Protection Act 1998 and the Freedom of Information Act 2000. www.informationcommissioner.gov.uk.

Advisory organisations and contact details

All of these organisations give advice to parents, and many are active in lobbying and campaigning as well.

ACE (Advisory Centre for Education)
Education Helpline 0808 800 5793. Exclusion information line 020 7704 9822. www.ace-ed.org
An independent education advice centre.

Audit Commission
Telephone 0800 502030. www.audit-commision.gov.uk

Connexions
Telephone 080 800132. www.connexions.gov.uk
Connexions is the government's support service for all young people aged 13 to 19 in England.

Contact a Family, 209–211 City Road, London EC1V 1JN.
Telephone 0808 8083555. www.cafamily.org
Contact a Family provides advice, information and support to all parents of disabled children including those with a specific and rare health condition.

Council for Disabled Children, 8 Wakley Street, London EC1V 1JN
Telephone 020 7843 6000. www.ncb.org.uk
Provides policy and practice information on a wide range of children's disability issues. Manages the National Parent Partnership Network and the Special Education Consortium

DfES Publications, PO Box 5050, Sherwood Park, Annesley, Nottingham NG15 0DJ. Telephone 0845 60 222 60. www.dfes.gov.uk/publications

DH Publications Orderline, PO Box 777, London SE1 6XH
Telephone 08701 555 455. dh@prolog.uk.com

Family Rights Group (FRG), The Print House, 18 Ashwin Street, London E8 3DL. Telephone 020 7923 2628. www.frg.org.uk
Provides advice and support for families whose children are involved with social services about the care and protection of children. They run a free telephone advice service 10am–12pm and 1.30–3.30pm each weekday on 0800 731 1696, and can advise on family support, child protection and related issues. They also have a number of advice sheets which can be downloaded directly from their website.

IPSEA (Independent Panel for Special Education Advice)
General enquiries 01394 380518. Helpline 0800 0184 4016. Tribunal Appeals 01394 384711. www.ipsea.org.uk
Provides free advice and support for parents whose children have SEN.

National Autistic Society (NAS), 393 City Road, London EC1V 1NG
General Helpline 0845 070 4004. Advocacy for Education Service 0845 070 4002. Head Office 020 7833 2299. www.nas.org.uk
Leading membership organisation and service provider for people with autism. Helpline has lists of local and regional autism groups in each area.

NAS Publications, Emotional, Units 2–3 Gales Gardens, Birbeck Street, London E2 0EJ. Telephone 020 7033 9237. naspublications@e-motional.org. www.nas.org.uk/pubs

PARIS (Public Autism Resource and Information Service)
www.info.autism.org.uk
An online database provided by NAS which gives details of autism-specific services across the UK.

Peach (Parents for the Early Intervention of Autism), The Brackens, London Road, Ascot, Berkshire, SL5 8BE. Telephone 01344 882248. www.peach.org.uk
Parent-led charity established to promote early behavioural intervention for young children with autism.

TreeHouse, Woodside Avenue, London, N10 3SA. Telephone 020 8815 5444. www.treehouse.org.uk
The national charity for autism education in the UK. Provides advice to parents looking to set up schools.

Other resources

Census 2001
www.statistics.gov.uk/census200
The information on this site allows you to calculate the likely numbers of children in your area. Go to 'Local Authority Profiles' and click the letter with which your authority's name starts. Click on 'population' and add up the totals in the first four rows to get the population of children under 20 in your authority in 2001.

Charity Commission, London Office: Harmsworth House, 13–15 Bouverie Street, London. EC4Y 8DP
Liverpool Office: 20 Kings Parade, Queens Dock, Liverpool L3 4DQ
Taunton Office: Woodfield House, Tangier, Taunton, Somerset TA1 4BL
Newport Office: 8th Floor, Clarence House, Clarence Place, Newport, South Wales NP19 7AA
For all general Charity Commission enquiries, call 0870 333 0123.
www.charity-commision.gov.uk

Health Service Ombudsman
www.ombudsman.org.uk
If you need to make a complaint about a UK government department or one of its agencies, or the NHS in England, ring the complaints Helpline 0845 015 4033 or e-mail phso.enquiries@ombudsman.org.uk, or make a complaint online. Or write to: The Parliamentary and Health Service Ombudsman, Millbank Tower, Millbank, London, SW1P 4QP

Local Government Ombudsman
www.lgo.org.uk
There are three Local Government Ombudsmen in England. Each of them deals with complaints from different parts of the country. To find out more you can contact the Adviceline, on 0845 602 1983. To order publications or copies of the Ombudsmen's reports, telephone the London office on 020 7217 4683, or send a publications order form.

NACVS (The National Association of Councils for Voluntary Service)
177 Arundel Street, Sheffield S1 2NU. Telephone 0114 278 6636.
www.nacvs.org.uk/
Helps to promote voluntary and community action by supporting its 350 member Councils for Voluntary Service in England and by acting as a national voice for the local voluntary and community sector.

NCVO (National Council for Voluntary Organisations)
Regent's Wharf, 8 All Saints Street, London N1 9RL. Switchboard 020 7713 616.
HelpDesk 0800 2 798 798. HelpDesk@ncvo-vol.org.uk. www.ncvo-vol.org.uk
NCVO works with and for the voluntary sector in England by providing information, advice and support and by representing the views of the sector to government and policy-makers.

Parent Partnership Network
8 Wakley Street London EC1V 7QE
Telephone 020 7843 6000. www.parentpartnership.org.uk
The website provides links to your local parent partnership service.

Special Educational Needs and Disability Tribunal (SENDIST)
Telephone 0870 241 2555. www.sendist.gov.uk
SENDIST annual reports have information broken down by each local authority – see www.sendist.gov/uk then click "About" then click "Our Annual Report" for the most recent.

Contact PACE

PACE is now the policy and campaigns tean of Treehouse, the national charity for autism education in the UK. PACE wants to hear from all parent campaigners who have used our Parent Handbook. We can put campaigners in touch with each other and communicate your experiences to national government.

PACE (Policy and Campaigns), TreeHouse, Woodside Avenue, London N10 3JA
Telephone 020 8815 5441.
Email handbook@treehouse.org.uk
For regular updates on government policy and parent campaigning, go to www.pace-uk.org.

List of abbreviations

ASD	autism spectrum disorder
CaF	Contact a Family
CAMHS	child and adolescent mental health services
CDC	Council for Disabled Children
DfES	Department for Education and Skills
DoH	Department of Health
EP	educational psychologist
LEA	local education authority
LGO	local government ombudsman
NAP-C	National Autism Plan for Children (National Autistic Society 2003b)
NAS	National Autistic Society
NSF	National Service Framework
OT	occupational therapist
PARIS	Public Autism Resource Information Service
PCT	primary care trust
PGR	parent governor representative
SEN	special educational needs
SENDIST	Special Educational Needs and Disability Tribunal
SLD	severe learning disability

Index